Pluralistic Sand-Tray Therapy

In this book, Fleet provides the first comprehensive guide to implementing sand-tray therapy within a pluralistic framework.

Pluralistic Sand-Tray Therapy offers several unique contributions to a theoretical understanding of the therapeutic process, including the dynamic phenomenological field incorporating the concept of phenomenological shift and the introduction to two sand-tray specific mechanisms that aid the therapeutic process by facilitating the client's discovery in a unique way. Theory is applied to practice with step-by-step detailed guidance on how to deliver effective pluralistic sand-tray therapy from the initial appointment to the end of therapy. Each theoretical concept and practical direction is supported by case study findings, including photographs taken during real sessions.

This book will be an essential text for academics and students of psychotherapy and counselling seeking to understand the impact and implementation of sand-tray therapy. It also offers a complete guide for practicing counsellors and psychotherapists, including arts and play therapists, who wish to use sand-tray therapy in their work.

Dr Doreen Fleet is a chartered psychologist (Counselling) with the BPS and became BACP accredited in 2007. She was a senior university lecturer and currently offers external postgraduate research supervision at the University of Chester. Doreen has consistently used creative ways of working throughout her teaching and counselling career.

Pluralistic Sand-Tray Therapy

Humanistic Principles for Working Creatively with Adult Clients

Doreen Fleet

Routledge
Taylor & Francis Group

LONDON AND NEW YORK

Cover image: © Doreen Fleet

First published 2023
by Routledge
4 Park Square, Milton Park, Abingdon, Oxon OX14 4RN

and by Routledge
605 Third Avenue, New York, NY 10158

Routledge is an imprint of the Taylor & Francis Group, an informa business

British Library Cataloguing-in-Publication Data
A catalogue record for this book is available from the British Library

Library of Congress Cataloging-in-Publication Data
Names: Fleet, Doreen, author.
Title: Pluralistic sand-tray therapy: humanistic principles for working creatively with adult clients / Doreen Fleet.
Description: Abingdon, Oxon; New York, NY: Routledge, 2022. |
Includes bibliographical references and index. |
Identifiers: LCCN 2022003701 | ISBN 9780367747749 (pbk) |
ISBN 9780367746117 (hbk) | ISBN 9781003158707 (ebk)
Subjects: LCSH: Play therapy. | Art therapy.
Classification: LCC RJ505.P6 F54 2022 |
DDC 618.92/891653–dc23/eng/20220318
LC record available at https://lccn.loc.gov/2022003701

ISBN: 978-0-367-74611-7 (hbk)
ISBN: 978-0-367-74774-9 (pbk)
ISBN: 978-1-003-15870-7 (ebk)

DOI: 10.4324/9781003158707

Typeset in Times New Roman
by Newgen Publishing UK

Contents

Chapter 1

Introduction

Sand and its symbolism

Human beings are fascinated by sand. Such fascination is apparent when observing people sitting on a beach wiggling their toes, pushing them into the sand or using their hands to sift, manipulate, and build with it spontaneously. Welland (2009) described how sand had a mysterious quality and a profound symbolism throughout history and many cultures. He views it as an enigmatic substance with a mysterious quality, "dry sand itself behaves eerily like a liquid, but wet sand behaves more like a solid" (Welland, 2009, p. 51). Dry or wet, it is a compelling substance, and touching and handling sand can bring a powerful tactile experience. It is a substance that is infinitely expressive and has been used by people to tell stories of the past and the future and to symbolise a constantly changing present (Welland, 2009).

Followers of Tibetan Tantric Buddhism create exquisite sand mandalas to express harmony and restore order, believing that these spiritual symbols provide healing and meditation guides (Welland, 2009, p. 219). The Sanskrit word "mandala" means circle, interpreted as "wheels within wheels" (Welland, 2009, p. 219). A Buddhist ceremony where a mandala created and then wiped away represents the view that life is transitory and impermanent, the truth that life and the world are constantly changing, constantly transitioning.

Jim Denevan, a contemporary sand artist, draws artwork in the sand at carefully chosen locations on beaches. He incorporates spirals and other simple geometrics to produce his artwork. Denevan (2009, www.jimdenevan. com) views the beach as a blank canvas and suggests that the sand-work symbolic process is a spiritual one, communicating "constant change": in a similar way to the Buddhist sand mandalas, there is an impermanence to Denevan's work, as the sand drawings usually exist for a few hours before the tide washes them away.

The sand work of both Tibetan Buddhists and sand artists is encapsulated in the quote,

One picture is worth ten thousand words.

DOI: 10.4324/9781003158707-1

This phrase is generally attributed to Fred R. Barnard, who wrote this when advertising in 1921 (Barnard, 1921). My view is that it is not only drawings in the sand that can hold profound symbolism but also objects placed into the sand, representing thoughts, emotions, behaviour, and unconscious material, creating a symbolic picture full of meaning for the person. Sand-tray therapy uses such symbolic objects, with the client placing them into a small sand tray and the therapist helping to facilitate the client's exploration and expression of their psychological and emotional distress.

> In most cases, all around the world, the margin between sea and land is defined by sand. Where sand is absent, there may be a hard cliff face and a raging sea, there is no softening between, no transition; where there is no sand, land and sea do battle. This could be an analogy for sand-tray therapy: the sand-tray described as the transition zone between the client's emotional/psychological distress and the healing process. With the help of the counsellor, the client may be able to work through their pain, by placing objects in the sand, which symbolize aspects of their experience relating to their issue/s.
>
> (Fleet, 2019, p. 1)

What is sand-tray therapy?

Sand-tray therapy is a therapeutic approach with the client selecting objects that represent their experience, arranging them into the sand tray. Kalff (2003) described how a client's experience is projected into the sand tray, being "transferred from the inner world to the outer world and made visible" (p. 9). The therapist helps the client explore their experience, and the approach adopted will be related to the therapist's theoretical orientation. The current theoretical literature on sand-tray therapy is predominantly Jungian sandplay (Kalff, 1971; Turner, 2005), composed of journal articles and books. Alongside this, a small volume of work produced by other authors from other orientations such as person-centred (Woodhouse, 2008), gestalt (Stevens, 2004), solution-focused therapy (SFT; Taylor, 2009), and the eclectic stance (Homeyer & Sweeney, 2011) exist. However, these books and articles almost entirely focus on delivering the therapy rather than understanding the theory related to the client's process.

When engaging with sand-tray therapy, clients often hold the objects as they talk or move them around the tray as they begin to express their thoughts and feelings. I have often supported clients to explore their issues related to their grief, despair, and hopelessness, and the "symbolic representation of these objects has helped them to explicitly communicate their deep pain" (Fleet, 2015, p. 16). At other times, existential issues emerge, and clients may begin to explore their mortality represented by the object/s. For some, the issue is fearful, yet as they begin to explore and express their fear using this creative

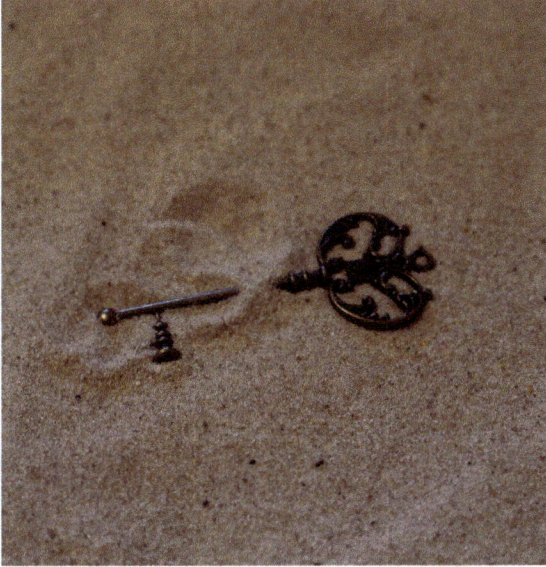

Image 1.1 Sand-tray is key to the client's process, decreasing their psychological and emotional distress.

(Fleet, 2019, cover page).

intervention, they can move to a place where acceptance, understanding, and meaning seem to result in the fear diminishing. Rothenberg (2011) appeared to offer a similar understanding by suggesting that creative thinking in sandplay (Kalff, 1980) is process-orientated, resulting in the person finding meaning in life, even when acknowledging that death is inevitable. In my work with my clients, it is as if they have found the *"key to unlocking their pain,"* and they become able to find their *"right"* words to express it (Image 1.1).

Some clients use the sand tray to symbolise the positive aspects of their life, such as happy memories or their coping mechanisms representing safety and self-protection. The physical and symbolic picture in the sand can reinforce the client's capacity to cope with a problematic issue. In addition, the same client may focus entirely on their pain in one session and on what they love about their life in another session or move back and forth in the same session. My belief is to stay alongside the client and help them lead, being free to set the agenda throughout each session.

Historical context

Nature has given us two ears, two eyes, and but one tongue – to the end that we should hear and see more than we speak.

(Socrates, Greek philosopher [470–399 BC])

Margaret Lowenfeld (1890–1973) was accepted as the pioneer of sand-tray therapy with children and introduced her approach, The World Technique (1979).

She believed that there was a necessity to supplement talking therapy with a visual medium, which the child could manipulate to aid their expression. Lowenfeld's approach was phenomenological, with her adopting the role of the "attentive observer" (Stevens, 2004), gently asking questions at the appropriate time without disrupting the process. This intervention gave the therapist additional cues to watch and hear the child play as they engaged with the sand tray.

Lowenfeld's motivation to incorporate sand tray into play therapy came from reading H.G. Wells' book, Floor Games (1911). Wells described how he often sat on the floor with his sons and played elaborate games using toys. Wells' behaviour was the catalyst for Lowenfeld to begin using trays with sand, water, and objects to guide the child to create a world picture. She stated how this was a valuable technique giving children a way of expressing their "ideas and feelings which won't go into words" (Lowenfeld, 1993, p. 4). She viewed the tactile nature of sand tray as a particular strength and the process of projection being significant to work through painful experience. Lowenfeld believed that "The World Technique" enabled the child to heal through play.

In 1954, Dora Kalff, a Jungian therapist, attended a lecture given by Lowenfeld and became interested in adopting this symbolic tool in therapy.

Kalff later adapted sand-tray work to incorporate archetypal content and symbolic processes and identified the core aim for the client to express conflicts that are still in the unconscious mind, naming this approach "sandplay" (Kalff, 1980), distinguishing it from Lowenfeld's work.

Contemporary literature on sand-tray therapy

Jungian sandplay predominates contemporary literature on sand-tray therapy and includes work with adult clients, children, and young people. Turner (2005) described how sandplay facilitates "transformation at the deepest levels of the psyche" (p. 695). The client expresses unconscious conflict using the sand tray, resulting in an innate move towards wholeness as the integration between their inner and external world occurs as they express their experience (Kalff, 1980; Turner, 2005). Ryce-Menuhin (1992) described how the symbolic picture presented in the sand could represent meanings that are not known or fully grasped by the client and the therapist; however, as the therapy progresses, the symbols act "as a bridge: the bridging of what is familiar to that which is strange. It relates the conscious to the unconscious, the literal to the abstract, the part to the whole" (p. 22). This visual, kinaesthetic, and metaphorical process aids the expressive communication of the client, facilitating the therapeutic process (Ryce-Menuhin, 1992).

The centre of the sand tray is highly significant in Jungian sandplay. Turner (2005) suggested that an object placed in the centre indicated an archetype of Self (Jung, 1971) that is activated and "pulls the psyche towards centering" (p. 258). Turner (2005) explained, "ultimately life is a journey to the centre ... a return to the source of one's being and a passage out of un-truth" (p. 259). Objects placed in the centre often occur towards the end of the sandplay process, and Turner (2005) argued that this indicates progression related to integrating aspects of the client's previously disconnected experience. Similarly, manipulating the sand, such as burying objects and digging them up, may indicate a new capacity to stay with initially overwhelming emotions.

Like Lowenfeld's approach, the concept of interpretation is a significant feature of Jungian sandplay. Ryce-Menuhin (1992) described how the therapist interprets the client's symbolic meaning when suitable in the sandplay process. He suggested how the symbolic interpretation raises the possibility of strengthening the client's ego; "the ego considers the interpretation revealed and can unite this with the self" (p. 89). The concept of archetypes is central to interpretation in sandplay. Like Freud (1920), Jung described the psyche as being made up of several parts. Jung labelled these "archetypes" (1971), including the Self, the Persona, the Shadow, the Mother, the Trickster. Each archetype is an inborn model of a person's behaviour and personality.

Jung encouraged his clients to "dialogue with these figures from the unconscious as if they were real people in the external world" (Storr, 1973, p. 13). Turner (2005) argued that sandplay is a medium that can access archetypal experience in the collective unconscious (Jung, 1971); inherited symbols of humankind, which not only have tremendous potential for the individual but also can contribute to global healing by increasing connection to all things.

However, there is an essential distinction between Lowenfeld and Turner's understanding and approach to interpretation. Lowenfeld (1979, 1993 "interpreted the child's Worlds before the end of treatment" (Turner, 2005, p. 694), viewing immediacy as essential to facilitate the client's expression of their thoughts and emotions.

Lowenfeld believed that this process helped release conflict and tension produced by discrepancies between the child's inner and outer realities (Turner, 2005, p. 695). In contrast, Kalff (1980, 2003) argued that a delayed interpretation was required to enable the client to "undergo transformation at the deepest levels of the psyche" (Turner, 2005, p. 695). Ryce-Menuhin (2015) described how "a silent observing companion" (p. 32) with a shared interpretation of the symbolism is effective when the time feels right. Sedgwick (2001) questioned interpretation in Jungian therapy, arguing how "practically speaking ...a client may not know what the therapist is talking about" (p. 65).

Turner (2005) adopted a similar stance stating, "no interpretation is made in Jungian sandplay" (p. 375) based on the rationale that the client is accessing their unconscious experience, and it takes time for that content and processes to become conscious. Turner believes the therapist needs to adopt an essentially non-verbal stance, with them practising containment "known as the free and protected space"(p. 135). The concept of containment, described as holding "the client's emerging unconscious material" (Turner, 1994, 2005, p. 3), creates a safe environment. However, a Jungian therapist who does not offer interpretation in a session is still likely to explore their interpretations and associated archetype symbols in clinical supervision to understand the client's process.

The question of "is therapist interpretation of a client's symbols in sand-tray therapy necessary?" would be answered with a resounding "no" from a humanistic therapist. Person-centred therapy (PCT) (Rogers, 1957), which is part of the humanistic tradition, views clients as having the innate capacity to solve their own problems.

Rogers (1951) identified the "actualising tendency" with the person having a genetic predisposition for growth in an ideal environment. Here, the therapist aims to offer the core conditions of unconditional positive regard, empathy, and congruency (Rogers, 1957; Merry, 1999).

Mearns and Thorne (1999) described how a congruent therapist would avoid "putting up a professional front or a personal facade" (p. 15), communicating that it is both permissible and desirable to be oneself. Offering unconditional positive regard is about offering the client total acceptance without judgement (Mearns & Thorne, 1999). Offering empathy involves accurately perceiving and tracking the client's feelings and personal meanings and communicating this understanding.

This stance argues that a therapist who acts on their interpretations of the client's process is motivated by their frame of reference, away from the client's experience (Axline, 1969). The risk is that therapist interpretation can impact the power balance and negatively affect the client's developing sense of autonomy and empowerment (Axline, 1969). Woodhouse (2008) used PCT sand tray with children, arguing that it was essential to stay alongside the client as they work with the sand tray, avoiding bringing preconceived assumptions into the therapeutic process. For example, an object of a dragon may mean fear to one client yet protection to another, so the therapist needs to work with the client's symbolism of the objects used instead of imposing their interpretation. Woodhouse (2008) placed significance on the core conditions, particularly empathy and unconditional positive regard, facilitating the child to feel valued, develop trust, and increase their awareness. She stated, "the child pours their process into the sand, they make a vivid picture of their inner dialogue and way of seeing the world" (Woodhouse, 2008, p. 32). Woodhouse (2008) used Polanyi's (1958) term of "indwelling," arguing how the therapist needs to indwell, entering the child's world as they experience themselves through the sand-tray process. However, a psychodynamic practitioner may criticise this view, suggesting how some clients are well defended and may not engage without direct intervention.

Also, a client may not be aware of a block; sometimes, the therapist can "see" something that the client cannot (Farber & Doolin, 2011).

The gestalt approach is also part of the humanistic tradition developed by Fritz Perls, Hefferline and Goodman, first published in the book *Gestalt Therapy* (1951). Stevens (2004) used sand tray as a "simple form of experimentation" (p. 18) in gestalt therapy. In line with PCT, Stevens viewed "organismic self-regulation" (Stevens, 2004, p. 2) as significant, enabling the client to move towards healing. Stevens has an affinity to Woodhouse's (2008) belief that sand-tray therapy is not about interpreting the client's experience or identifying universal symbols. However, it differs from PCT as the gestalt therapist takes a more active approach (Stevens, 2004); they show curiosity about the client's sand display and communicate this by asking questions and becoming engaged in the client's process.

Stevens (2004) used a sand tray with adult clients and children and described how some adults are surprised when offered this way of working in therapy. Her motivation for offering this intervention comes when an adult is experiencing some block in the therapeutic process, such blocks arising from an adult's tendency to intellectualise. Stevens (2004) argued how the sand-tray intervention helps adult clients bypass their resistance to "creative play," "it is though we came around the backdoor and caught ourselves out" (p. 11). Stevens viewed this as a strength, helping the adult to communicate in a more open, spontaneous, and creative manner, freeing them from the confines of their tendency to intellectualise.

A small volume of literature on integrating sand tray to SFT is available (Taylor, 2009). Taylor indicated that this way of working could produce an "empowering and brief experiential therapeutic journey" (2009, p. 56) for clients. This approach attempts to help the client move their attention away from a problem by identifying their strengths and developing their coping skills. The sessions tend to be structured, which contrasts with PCT; the client is free to set the agenda. An SFT therapist will incorporate questions about exceptions to the problem, scaling a problem and the "miracle question" (Macdonald, 2007). Scaling a problem involves the client rating their problem on a scale (1–10 or 1–100) to indicate how significant it is to them at that time.

The miracle question is a common strategy in SFT, helping the client think creatively and move their attention away from the problem by imagining that the problem has gone by some miracle, facilitating the client to visualise how that would be. Taylor (2009) suggested that the therapist could ask the client to create a picture in the sand of how their world would look if the problem did not exist.

Homeyer and Sweeney (2011) described their approach to sand tray as eclectic (p. 4). They discussed how they include ways of working from other orientations, including Rational-Emotive Behaviour Therapy (Ellis, 2008), SFT (de Shazer et al., 2007), and psychodynamic/Jungian concepts such as defences. However, Patterson (1989) criticised the eclectic approach, arguing how combining limited methods and strategies with little attention to theory is inadequate. However, Homeyer and Sweeney (2011) take a different stance on this, focusing on strategies from different approaches, and incorporate some theoretical concepts such as defences, intrapsychic issues, and projection in their description of their eclectic approach.

The single modalities and approaches to sand tray discussed so far have specific benefits. Except for Homeyer and Sweeney's (2011) eclectic approach, they remain separate, standing alone as single orientations and not drawing upon strengths from other stances. In contrast, the Pluralistic approach (Cooper & McLeod, 2007; McLeod, 2015; Cooper & Dryden, 2016; Cooper & McLeod, 2011; McLeod, 2018), which is relatively new within the counselling field, does draw on the strengths of other orientations to work creatively in therapy to ensure that each client receives the therapy that is suited to them (Cooper & McLeod, 2011).

The stance of drawing on different orientations contrasts with "monism" based on the understanding that there is a definitive answer to every question arguing against the assumption that there is a "best way" of working in therapy (Cooper & McLeod, 2011). Cooper and Dryden (2016) stated: "different understandings are useful for different clients at different points in time" (p. 3). The central aim of pluralistic therapy is that "therapists should work closely with their clients to decide on how the work should proceed" (Cooper & McLeod, 2011, p. 6).

Until my case study research (Fleet, 2019), which established a pluralistic framework of sand-tray therapy, there was a gap in the literature on using sand tray from a pluralistic standpoint. Furthermore, apart from Jungian sandplay, there is limited literature on using sand tray with adult clients. This book aims to inform the reader of the theoretical therapeutic process and guidance on conducting pluralistic sand-tray therapy with adult clients.

The book will explore how the therapist can take a collaborative approach, including the client in a shared decision-making creative process by engaging in dialogical conversation (McLeod, 2018) throughout therapy. The turn-taking and the sharing of ideas from both client and therapist affirm the client and utilise the therapist's knowledge (Cooper & McLeod 2007). McLeod (2018) suggested that this process involves purposeful conversation, described as "metacommunication." He stated, "the act of standing back from the on-going flow of communication, reflecting on (or inviting reflection on) the intentions and/ or reactions of the speaker and/or listener" (p. 18) likened to metacommunication. However, it is more of a general strategy aiding collaboration.

Other processes, including goal setting, assessment, and feedback, are also significant in the pluralistic approach that "cultivates a client's agency" (McLeod & McLeod, 2016, p. 16).

The various elements of the pluralistic approach will be a theme throughout the book, aiming to demonstrate how this new framework is fundamentally pluralistic whilst based on humanistic principles for working creatively with adult clients.

All clients who engaged in the case study research (Fleet, 2019) [Ethical approval granted]) referred to in this book gave informed consent to publish their experience and photographs of their sand displays and are anonymised to protect their identities.

This book is derived in part from a PhD study by Fleet, D. (2019). *Transformation hidden in the sand: Developing a theoretical framework using a sand-tray intervention with adult clients.* Doctoral thesis. Staffordshire University. Stoke-on-Trent. Available from Ethos ST
ORE – Staffordshire Online Repository. https://eprints.staffs.ac.uk/id/eprint/5763

In addition, this book is derived in part from an article in *Journal of Creativity in Mental Health* 14/6/21, copyright Taylor & Francis, available online: www.tandfonlinecom/ DOI 10.1080/15401383.2021.1936738

References

Axline, V. (1969). *Play therapy.* New York: Ballantine.

Barnard, F. R. (1921). *One look is worth a thousand words (p. 96).* Printers Ink

Cooper, M., & Dryden, W. (2016). *The handbook of pluralistic counselling and psychotherapy.* London: Sage.

Cooper, M., & McLeod, J. (2007). A pluralistic framework for counselling and psychotherapy: Implications for research. *Counselling and Psychotherapy Research, 7*(3), 135–143. Retrieved from http://eprints.cdlr.strath.ac.uk/5213/

Cooper, M., & McLeod, J. (2011). *Pluralistic counselling and psychotherapy.* London: Sage.

Denevan, J. (2009). Home page. www.jimdenevan.com Retrieved October 2020.

de Shazer, S., Berg, I. K., Lipchik, E., Nunnally, E., Molnar, A., Gingerich, W., & Weiner-Davis, M. (1986). Brief therapy: Focused solution development. *Family Process, 25,* 207–22.

de Shazer, S., Dolan, Y., Korman, H., Trepper, T., McCollum, E., & Berg, I. K. (2007). *More than miracles the state of the art solution-focused brief therapy.* Binghamton, NY: Hawthorne.

Ellis, A. (2008). Rational emotive behavior therapy. In R. Corsini & D. Wedding (Eds.), *Current psychotherapies* (8th ed.; pp. 187–222). Belmont, CA: Thomson.

Farber, B., & Doolin, E. M. (2011). Positive regard. *Psychotherapy, 48*(1), 58–64. https://doi.org/10.10.37/a0022141

Fleet, D. (2015, Spring). Beyond Words: Creative words have an established evidence base when working with children and young people but why are they not more widely used when counselling adults? *Private Practice* (pp. 14–17). British Association for Counselling and Psychotherapy.

Fleet, D. (2019). *Transformation hidden in the sand: Developing a theoretical framework using a sand-tray intervention with adult clients.* Doctoral thesis. Staffordshire

University. Stoke-on-Trent. Available from Ethos STORE – Staffordshire Online Repository. https://eprints.staffs.ac.uk/id/eprint/5763

Fleet, D., Reeves, A., Burton, A., & DasGupta, M. P. (2021). Transformation hidden in the sand: A pluralistic theoretical framework using sand-tray with adult clients. First published online (14 June, 2021). *Journal of Creativity in Mental Health.* https://doi.org/10.1080/15401383.2021.1936738

Freud, S. (1920). *A general introduction to psychoanalysis.* New York: PDF Books World. www.pdfbooksworld.com

Homeyer, L., & Sweeney, D. (2011). *Sandtray therapy: A practical manual* (2nd ed.). London: Routledge.

Jung, C. G. (1971). The archetypes and the collective unconscious. In H. Read, M. Fordham, G. Adler, & W. McGuire (Eds.), (R. F. C. Hull, Trans.), *Collected works of C. G. Jung* (Vol. 9.1). Princeton, NJ: Princeton University Press. (Original work published in 1934.)

Kalff, D. (1971). *Sandplay: Mirror of a child's psyche.* San Francisco, CA: C. G. Jung Institute.

Kalff, D. (1980). *Sandplay: A psychotherapeutic approach to the psyche.* Santa Monica, CA: Sigo Press.

Kalff, D. (2003). *Sandplay: A psychotherapeutic approach to the psyche.* Cloverdale, CA: Temenos Press.

Lowenfeld, M. (1979). *The world technique.* London: Allen & Unwin.

Lowenfeld. M. (1993). *Understanding children's sandplay: Lowenfeld's world technique.* Great Britain: Antony Rowe Ltd.

Macdonald, A. (2007). *Solution-focused therapy: Theory, research & practice.* London: Sage.

McLeod, J. (2015). A pluralistic framework for counselling and psychotherapy practice: Implications for therapist training and development. *E-Journal for biopsychosoziale dialoge in psychtherapie, supervision und beratung.* Retrieved from www.resonanzen-journal.org

McLeod, J. (2018). *Pluralistic therapy: Distinctive features.* London: Routledge, Taylor & Francis Group.

McLeod, J., & McLeod, J. (2016). Assessment and formulation in pluralistic counselling and psychotherapy. In M. Cooper & W. Dryden (Eds.), *The handbook of pluralistic counselling and psychotherapy* (pp. 15–27). London: Sage.

Mearns, D., & Thorne, B. (1999). *Person-centred counselling in action* (2nd ed.). In W. Dryden (Ed.). London: Sage Publications.

Merry, T. (1999; 2002). *Learning and being in person-centred counselling.* Ross-on-Wye: PCCS Books.

Patterson, C. H. (1989). Eclecticism in psychotherapy: Is integration possible? *Psychotherapy, 26,* 157–161.

Perls, F., Hefferline, R., & Goodman, P. (1951). *Gestalt therapy: Excitement and growth in the human personality.* Gouldsboro, ME: Gestalt Journal Press.

Polanyi's. (1958). *Personal knowledge: Towards a post-critical philosophy.* Chicago, IL: University of Chicago Press.

Rogers, C. R. (1951). *Client-centered therapy: Its current practice, implications and theory.* London: Constable.

Rogers, C. R. (1957). The necessary and sufficient conditions of therapeutic personality change. *Journal of Consulting Psychology, 21,* 95–103.

Rothenberg, A. (2011). *Janusian processes*. In M. A Runco & S. R Pritzker (Eds.), Encyclopedia of creativity (pp. 103–108). San Diego, CA: Academic Press.

Ryce-Menuhin. (1992). *Jungian sandplay: The wonderful therapy*. New York: Routledge, Taylor & Francis Group.

Sedgwick, D. (2001). *Introduction to Jungian psychotherapy: The therapeutic relationship*. East Sussex: Brunner-Routledge, Taylor & Francis Group.

Stevens, C. (2004). Playing in the sand. *The British Gestalt Journal, 13*(1), 18–23.

Storr, A. (1973). *Jung*. London: Fontana Press.

Taylor, E. R. (2009). Sandtray and solution-focused therapy. *International Journal of Play Therapy, 18*(1), 56–68.

Turner, B. (1994). Symbolic process and the role of the therapist in sand-play. *Journal of Sandplay Therapy, 3*(2), 84–95.

Turner, B. A. (2005). *The handbook of sandplay therapy*. Cloverdale, California: Temenos Press.

Welland, M. (2009). *Sand: The never-ending story*. Berkeley: University of California Press.

Wells, H. G. (1911). *Floor Games*. Chicago, UK: Frank Palmer.

Woodhouse, J. (2008). SANDPLAY: Growing ground in person-centred play therapy. In S. Keys & T. Walshaw (Eds.), *Person-centred work with children and young people: UK practitioner perspectives* (pp. 29–38). Ross-on-Wye: PCCS Books.

Chapter 2

Introducing the pluralistic theoretical framework

No panacea to restoration

(Adapted from Fleet, 2019, p. 36)

The pluralistic approach is collaborative, flexible, and creative, aiming to fit the individual client's goals and expectations for therapy. Based on the rationale that one method is unlikely to suit all clients, this stance is conducive to the belief that people are unique and want different things from therapy (Cooper & McLeod, 2007).

The multiple case study research (Fleet, 2019) underpinning this book's focus established a pluralistic theoretical framework of sand-tray therapy with adult clients (Figure 2.1).

The framework comprises various elements of the phenomenological field relating to the client's intra-psychic experience that incorporates aspects of phenomenological shift, phenomenological flux, and pre-phenomenological process, which all originate from the foundation of the model. Reber's (1985) definition of the term intra-psychic is "anything assumed to arise or take place within the mind … intra-psychic conflicts refer to conflicts between beliefs, needs or desires" (p. 372). The argument is that sand-tray therapy can help access "deeper intrapsychic issues … more thoroughly and more rapidly" (Homeyer & Sweeney, 2011, p. 11), facilitating the processing of inner disturbance such as anxiety.

In addition to the elements of the framework already referred to above, there are two sand-tray specific mechanisms of phenomenological anchor and phenomenological hook that facilitate the therapeutic process and originate from the model's foundation.

The foundation of the framework

The foundation of the framework consists of three components: sand tray, pluralistic, and symbolism.

DOI: 10.4324/9781003158707-2

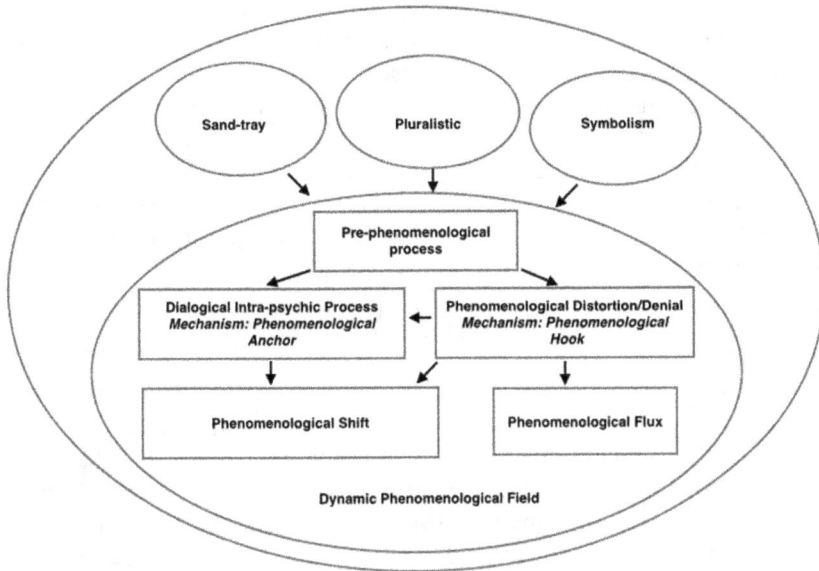

Figure 2.1 The pluralistic theoretical framework.
Adapted from Fleet (2019, p. 144).

Sand-tray component

The sand tray is not simply a therapeutic tool to be used as an addition to verbal communication but is more significant and integral to the therapeutic process. In this theoretical model, the sand tray described as a "metaphorical experiential theatre" serves as a stage where clients work with the objects representing their intra-psychic, inter-relational, and cultural/spiritual experiences by creating a physical picture in the sand (Fleet, 2019; Fleet et al., 2021).

This metaphor was adapted from Verhofstadt-Deneve et al. (2004), who used this metaphor in psychodrama to describe the psychodramatic "social atom method" when working with children in play therapy, using puppets and a blanket spread on the floor. The blanket served as a stage for the child to represent significant people in their life. Two therapists work with the children; the first, named "The Director," asks exploratory questions, and the second is "The Co-director" who aims to express the child's images, feelings, and thoughts. In this type of play therapy, the child called "The Protagonist"; the meaning resembling its use in the theatre is the leading character in a "play."

In pluralistic sand-tray therapy, the client is "The Director" of the "play." It is they who select the objects to represent their experience related to the issue explored (Fleet, 2019; Fleet et al., 2021). Additionally, they establish the general content, or the "act" of the "play," as they set the agenda of each session concerning what aspect of their experience they will focus on and symbolise with the objects. Unlike Verhofstadt-Deneve et al. method, the therapist has a more fluent role, sometimes being the empathic listener, offering the core conditions of empathy, unconditional positive regard, and congruency (Rogers, 1957; Mearns & Thorne, 1999; Merry, 2002).

The therapist will also paraphrase, putting what the client says in their own words (Steward, 2013) and reflect their thoughts, feelings, and body language enabling the client to feel understood and their thoughts and feelings accepted to communicate respect.

At other times, the therapist will take the role of "The Co-director" (Fleet, 2019; Fleet et al., 2021) of the "play" by asking Socratic questions (Padesky, 1993), making suggestions, offering challenges, and facilitating purposeful dialogue (McLeod, 2018). Padesky (1993) established the Socratic method used in therapy, and Socratic questions used in Cognitive Behavioural Therapy (CBT) help a client in guided discovery. Padesky described how a good Socratic question helps the client explore what they do not say and helps them move "from the concrete to the abstract" (Padesky, 1993, p. 2). An example used by Padesky to emphasise this skill is "What do you know now that you didn't know then?" (1993, p. 1). Kennerley (2007) described how she might ask a client, "What can you see in your mind's eye?" or "Can you tell me more about what's happening for you right now? (p. 23), which helps a client go further in their exploration.

Pluralistic component

The second component of the framework's foundation is pluralistic, which is central to the theoretical understanding of the counselling process and has practical application when adopting this approach to sand-tray work.

The pluralistic approach, initially established by Cooper and McLeod (2007), is founded on humanistic principles as it emphasises the client being an active agent of change (Cooper & McLeod, 2011). This stance acknowledges and values the client's autonomy by respecting their unique way of being (Cooper & McLeod, 2011). Cooper and McLeod (2011) described how "both James (1996) and McLellan (1995) suggest that pluralism may essentially be synonymous with humanism" (p. 17).

Cooper and McLeod (2007) advocated working collaboratively with the client, including them in shared decision-making and facilitating them to participate in a dialogical conversation, helping them move towards healing. McLeod (2018) stated how such dialogue between client and therapist is a "helpful and healing experience in itself" (p. 49). The sharing of ideas from both parties affirms the client's input and utilises the therapist's knowledge (Cooper & McLeod, 2007).

McLeod (2018) suggested that this type of dialogue is "metacommunication," which he described as "the act of standing back from the on-going flow of conversation, reflecting on (or inviting reflection on) the intentions and/or reactions of the speaker and/or listener" (p. 83). The aim is to acknowledge that the client has a valuable contribution, with the therapist remaining open to being corrected by them.

Such dialogical conversation occurs in the first meeting with the client to establish what they want from therapy, and a discussion will take place to decide how they may achieve that (Cooper & McLeod, 2011). The two-way conversation will involve identifying the goals, tasks, and methods of the therapy. McLeod (2018) discussed "goal setting" in pluralistic therapy as a flexible term, involving a client setting a concrete goal or having a "looser, more open goal for therapy." A concrete goal may involve a client needing a strategy to cope with their anxiety. Whereas a client may communicate a looser goal in that, they just want to feel happier.

When a goal emerges during therapy, a return to goal setting and purposeful dialogue at that time could be helpful in order to meet the client's expectations.

The collaborative approach in pluralistic therapy draws on the strengths of both client and therapist. It would be unhelpful for therapists to "ignore their own knowledge, experience and expertise when it comes to identifying tasks and methods for therapy" (Cooper & McLeod, 2007, p. 12). At times, a therapist will have specific knowledge of what may be helpful for a client that the client may not be aware of. For example, a client experiencing panic attacks may benefit from a relaxation technique facilitated by the therapist in therapy; the client outside of therapy can then practise this strategy when they become aware that their anxiety is beginning to build. Ongoing purposeful discussion during therapy sessions can focus on how helpful this strategy is for the client and signpost anything that needs to change.

Case study: Jackie

Jackie took part in the case study research (Fleet, 2019) and received six sessions of pluralistic sand-tray therapy. Her presenting problem was one of anxiety, and in the assessment session, she described being in a relationship with a married man who had left his wife so he could move in with Jackie. Although she was happy with her new partner, she was fearful that his family might persuade him to leave her and go back to them, leaving Jackie alone again.

Jackie was clear about her expectations of therapy, stating, "*I want to explore my feelings and find some peace with a more structured vision for my future*" (Fleet, 2019, p. 126). We discussed how talking about her thoughts and feelings relating to her fear that her partner may leave her might help, and she was happy to use the sand tray to do this. The following purposeful dialogue took place between her and me:

DOREEN: *"So you know when you said you would like to have peace and a more structured vision for the future ... how do you think that may look if you had that?"*

JACKIE: *"Erm ... not sure ... either be with him and it be less fraught and some consistency that he is there for the long haul ... or end it and just move on."*

DOREEN: *"Ok ... ay, so it sounds like you have a decision to make?"*

JACKIE: *"Suppose ... but I do want to be with him ... don't want him to go back to her."*

DOREEN: *"Hopefully, I can help you when using the sand tray to help you unpack all of that."*

JACKIE: *"But ... I avoid my feelings ... you need to be aware of that!"*

DOREEN: *"Sounds like you want me to be quite directive in terms of helping you to express your feelings."*

JACKIE: *"Yeah ... don't let me off the hook ... I'm very good at avoiding."*

DOREEN: *"That is helpful for me to know how you want me to work and that challenge and maybe some probing questions are going to be important in the sessions?"*

JACKIE: *"Yes ... don't just want you to sit there and nod ... want you to be active ... be in it with me ... yes ask me questions."*

(Fleet, 2019, pp. 126–127)

This purposeful two-way dialogue began when I asked the Socratic question of how her life might look if she had peace of mind. This question enabled Jackie to "stand back" and reflect on her hope and expectations of therapy. Furthermore, we had a good starting point on what might be a block for her in the therapeutic process, with her describing her tendency to avoid her feelings, providing a good strategy of asking probing questions to help her stay with her feelings.

This collaborative process was evident throughout Jackie's therapy, with shared decision making and turn taking being a consistent feature.

Case study: Grace

Grace was a married woman with two small children. She worked two days a week, with the rest of her time devoted to looking after the children and running the household. Her presenting issue was a relationship problem involving her anxiety surrounding her husband's heavy alcohol consumption. In the first three sessions, Grace had placed objects relating to her family into the centre of the sand and then selected an object to represent her, placing it next to the objects of her children. Throughout the first three sessions, she talked from the position of her family members in an interpersonal encounter, avoiding her feelings relating to her anxiety. An example of purposeful conversation midway through therapy occurred in the fourth therapy session:

I was thinking about your previous sessions, with you beginning by placing objects representing your family into the sand and was wondering how it would be to begin by choosing an object which represents you and place that in the centre first?

(Fleet, 2019, p. 156)

Grace responded to this challenge:

GRACE: *"Yeah ... a different way."*
DOREEN: *"What do you think by beginning the session that way might do?"* [Socratic question]
GRACE: *"For a start, I will have to focus on me instead of everyone else all the time."*
DOREEN: *"Yes ... it comes across how much you care about everyone else."*
GRACE: *"Okay...I'll do it."*

(Fleet, 2019, p. 156)

Grace decided to accept this suggestion that helped her realise that she needed to focus on her thoughts and feelings concerning her anxiety. She placed an object of a young female standing on a plinth (Image 2.1) into the middle of the sand-tray stating, *"this is me ... my perfect self"* and began to explore her

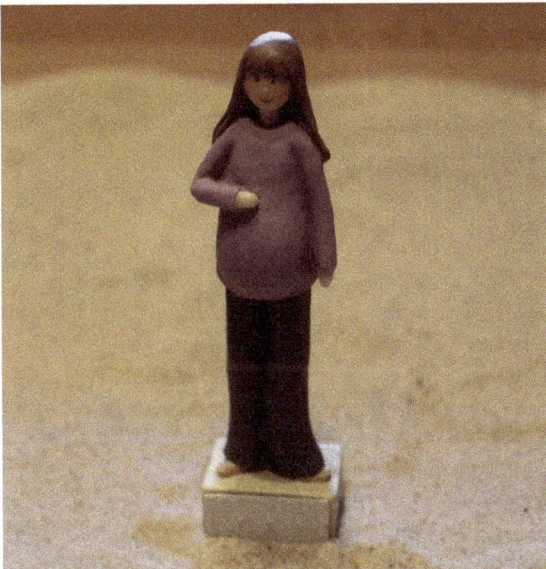

Image 2.1 Grace's perfectionist self.
(Fleet, 2019, p. 231).

perfectionist tendency, "*I worry so much if things are not one hundred per cent perfect*" (Fleet, 2019, p. 231).

Further along in this session, Grace concluded that she needed to learn that things cannot always be perfect. She did not want her children to become perfectionists like her, so she needed to work on her perfectionism that often caused her anxiety.

Another aspect the pluralistic approach views as significant, which "cultivates a client's agency" (McLeod & McLeod, 2016, p. 16), is assessment and feedback. Assessment and feedback also provide signposts of which ideas or theoretical perspectives may be helpful to meet the client's needs. Assessments may involve short or longer questionnaires such as the "Clinical Outcomes in Routine Evaluation" (Twigg & McInnes, 2010). The short CORE-10 questionnaire has ten items to measure psychological distress and is used routinely within counselling (Barkham et al., 2013). This measure used before therapy took place and compared with a post-therapy questionnaire once therapy has completed.

In addition, qualitative feedback can be obtained so the client can offer their unique perspective on their progress and their perceived usefulness of the therapy. However, whatever the measure used, the pluralistic approach takes every opportunity to engage the client in purposeful dialogue to help them reflect on their experience.

Case study: Shirley

In the initial appointment, Shirley's presenting issues were anxiety and panic attacks, which she said were having a negative impact on her life. She identified two goals for therapy: to manage her anxiety and panic attacks and talk about some difficult things she had not spoken of before. The following purposeful conversation took place near the end of the assessment session:

DOREEN: "*So you said you wanted to manage your anxiety.*"

SHIRLEY: "*Yes.*"

DOREEN: "*Well sometimes when you combine the breathing with imagination it can work well as a strategy.*"

SHIRLEY: "*How do you do that?*"

DOREEN: "*When you feel your panic building, where in your body … do you feel the anxiety?*"

SHIRLEY: "*In my chest* (put her hand on her chest)."

DOREEN: "(Mirrored body language, hand on chest) *When you feel the anxiety here … does a colour come to mind?*"

SHIRLEY: "*Red … yes red.*"

DOREEN: "*Okay … so if you can feel the opposite of that anxious feeling … what calm colour comes up for you?*"

SHIRLEY: "*Light blue.*"

DOREEN: *"So the next time you feel the panic and anxiety begin to build, you could imagine the red colour in your chest, and see and feel yourself breathing out the red anxiety and breathing in the calm blue colour and keep repeating it until the anxiety is gone along with the red and you are breathing in light blue and breathing out light blue."*

SHIRLEY: *"That sounds good I will do that."*

DOREEN: *"Would you like me to show you this at the end of the session?"*

SHIRLEY: *"Yes ... think that would be good."*

DOREEN: *"Okay sounds like a good idea ... let's see if it works."*

(Fleet, 2019, p. 154)

Although the initial idea of the relaxation strategy came from me as therapist, Shirley needed to be part of that process, and in deciding whether this was something, she wanted to try to manage her panic attacks. The goal of "wanting to speak about some difficult things she had not said before" was the focus of the sand-tray sessions, with her using the symbolic objects to explore her experience and speak out loud what she needed to. This combination worked well for Shirley, with her progress demonstrated in her final sand display (Image 3.2), representing her managing her panic and having a more positive outlook for her future. Her qualitative feedback on her experience of the sand-tray therapy was positive, and there was improvement in her CORE-10 scores (Figure 2.2).

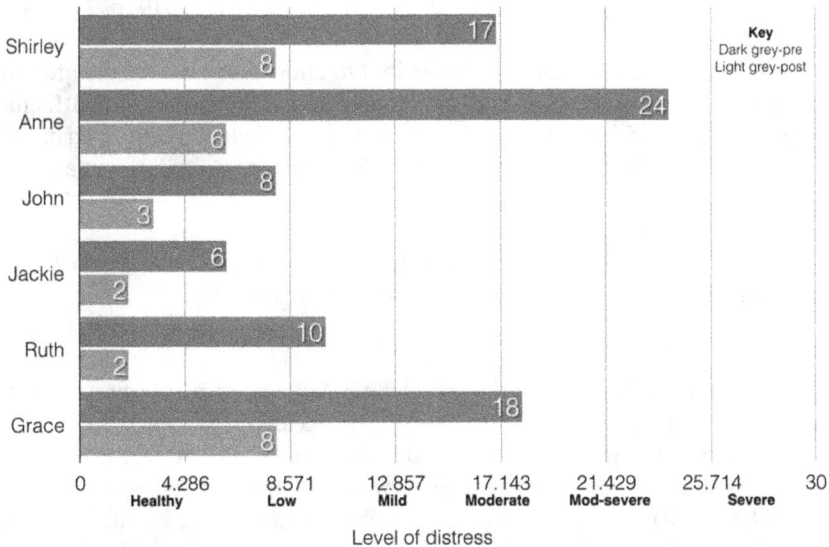

Figure 2.2 Graph of pre- and post-CORE-10 scores.
(Adapted from Fleet, 2019. p. 241).

The six clients who engaged in the case study all agreed to complete a CORE-10 pre- and post-questionnaire, and all showed improvement in the clinical scores after completing pluralistic sand-tray therapy, demonstrating a decrease in their level of distress (Figure 2.2).

Purposeful conversations can also occur at the end of each sand-tray therapy session focusing on the feedback from the client. At the end of the final session, the client asked to reflect on the whole of the therapy will give a further opportunity to voice their perspectives on whether they found the sand-tray therapy helpful. The clients in the case study stated:

SHIRLEY: *"Very helpful. It was useful to talk about why I have always felt so scared."*

ANNE: *"Things seemed hopeless at first. It helped me tremendously in exploring my inner feelings which I previously found hard to talk about."*

JOHN: *"In the first session I found myself crying, a good piece of closure."*

JACKIE: *"With you probing in the right areas helped me go deeper and to go with my feelings. The object being in front of you ... which you can't ignore. It helped me in evaluation of my stuff in such a fresh way."*

RUTH: *"It's a new experience using sand-tray and I have felt comfortable using it. It has given me visual not just verbal interaction. Helped me talk about things from my past, put that to bed now."*

GRACE: *"Helped me think about what I need to do, just so sad. Should I stay with him? Got a lot to think about. It was better than expected, it helped me to focus on my feelings and thoughts and see them clearly."*

(Fleet, 2019, p. 242–247)

In the final session, the client can be invited to choose an object/s they found most significant throughout sand-tray therapy, and the therapist can facilitate a discussion on how the significant object/s had helped them in terms of progression with their issue. For example, Anne placed an older woman in a wheelchair and a key into the sand stating:

> The old lady in the wheelchair was like the first of the early ones which I would say was the most significant...but now it is this key.

(Fleet, 2019, p. 118)

The object of the woman in the wheelchair Anne used in the first session had represented her worst fear that her severe accident may result in her not being able to walk. Although Anne could still walk by the end of therapy, her injured leg was shorter than the other, and she was not as physically able as before the accident happened. In later therapy sessions, Anne began to accept that although she had limitations and had to give up activities like dancing, she had other things to look forward to, and in the final session, she had a much more positive frame of mind, which she symbolised with the key object.

The dialogical conversation on the two objects focused on how Anne had changed, not only regarding her emotions, which she had freely expressed, but also regarding her thoughts and outlook for her future.

Purposeful discussion at the end of therapy can also focus on clinical scores such as pre- and post-CORE-10 scores indicating any improvement or not in the clients' levels of distress.

Symbolism component

The symbolism component refers to the objects selected by the client to represent their experience in sand-tray therapy. The definition of the word symbolism is "the use of symbols to represent ideas or qualities" (Hawker, 2006, p. 710). In sand-tray therapy, the objects act as physical symbols, representing a client's inner-experience (the phenomenological), personal history, personal relationships, and wider social and cultural experience, aiding interpersonal and intra-psychic processing.

Anne placed an object of a demon monster (Image 2.2) in the sand tray, which symbolised her hatred of being dependent on others since her accident.

Anne was a fiercely independent woman, yet her accident, resulting in a compound fracture to her femur, compromised her self-concept, leaving her physically dependent on others. In session 1, Anne described how she had

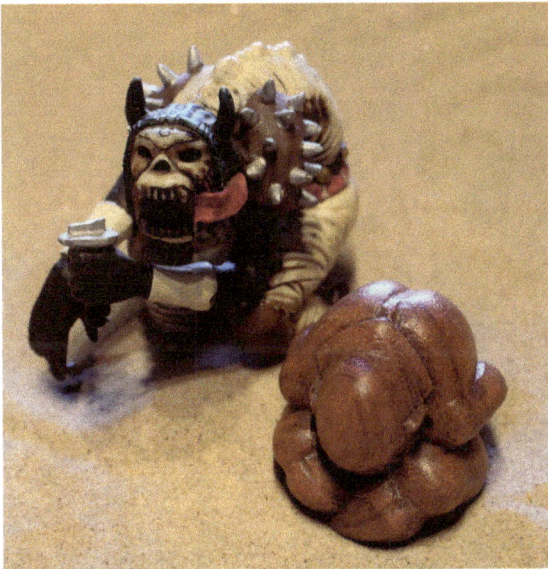

Image 2.2 Anne's demon monster object representing her hate of dependency.
(Fleet, 2019, p. 178).

never been dependent on anyone before her accident, and now that she had to be, she hated it.

Throughout this session, Anne expressed her frustration of relying on others and her distress related to her perceived loss of being an independent woman. The demon monster object represented her loss, and she expressed this in a powerfully emotive way.

Anne also explored an aspect of her personal history in a particular session, selecting an object of a young girl and laying it face down in the sand, symbolising her younger self. She described how as a spoilt child, she had temper tantrums if she did not get her own way. Together we worked with this symbolism, and Anne explored her younger self, connecting this aspect to herself as an adult. She began to realise that she still had temper tantrums even as an adult if she did not get her own way but expressed them differently by being selfish and raising her voice to her partner when he disagreed. This exploration resulted in her trying to change her behaviour, aiming to take a more adult attitude when communicating with him.

Shirley selected an object of a Buddha in her third session that represented her spiritual side (Image 2.3):

> *Yeah, the Buddha … if I could just bring this peace and* (picked up the heart from the basket and examined it closely) … *these broken lines inside*

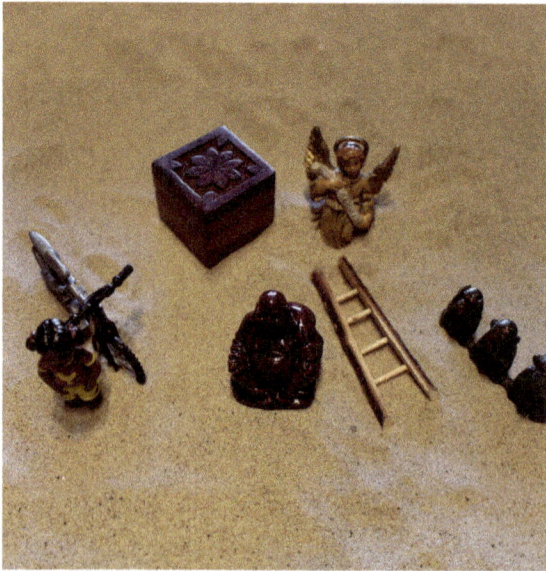

Image 2.3 Buddha object, Shirley's spiritual symbol.
(Fleet, 2019, p. 165).

it … all this self-doubt … if I don't blame myself … it could be the key to stopping the negative thoughts.

(Fleet, 2019, p. 167)

Shirley explored this spiritual symbol that helped her contemplate the possibility of her taking action. She aimed to stop her negative thoughts and her tendency to self-blame, and she began to acknowledge her need for calm and self-compassion, "*If … like … I could just bring that calmness*" (Fleet, 2019, p. 168). Here, she expressed her agency in how she could progress in terms of her panic. This understanding reinforced by the empathic reflection of "*It seems you know how you want to change to help you manage your panic*" (Fleet, 2019, p. 168) acknowledged Shirley's perception of how she could move towards healing.

References

Barkham, M., Bewick, B., Mullin, T., Gilbody, S., Connell, J., Cahill, J., Mellor-Clark, J., Richards, D., Unsworth G., & Evans, C. (2013). The CORE-10: A short measure of psychological distress for routine use in the psychological therapies. *Counselling and Psychotherapy Research*, *13*(1), 1–13. Retrieved from https://doi.org/10.1080/14733145.2012.729069

Cooper, M., & McLeod, J. (2007). A pluralistic framework for counselling and psychotherapy: Implications for research. *Counselling and Psychotherapy Research*, *7*(3), 135–143. Retrieved from http://eprints.cdlr.strath.ac.uk/5213/

Cooper, M., & McLeod, J. (2011). *Pluralistic counselling and psychotherapy*. London: Sage.

Fleet, D. (2019). *Transformation hidden in the sand: Developing a theoretical framework using a sand-tray intervention with adult clients*. Doctoral thesis. Staffordshire University. Stoke-on-Trent. Available from Ethos STORE – Staffordshire Online Repository. https://eprints.staffs.ac.uk/id/eprint/5763

Fleet, D., & Reeves, A., & Burton, A., & DasGupta, M. P. (2021). Transformation hidden in the sand: A pluralistic theoretical framework using sand-tray with adult clients. First published online (14 June 2021). *Journal of Creativity in Mental Health*. https://doi.org/10.1080/15401383.2021.1936738

Hawker, S. (2006). *Little Oxford English Dictionary* (9th ed.). Oxford: Oxford University Press.

Homeyer, L. E., & Sweeney, D. S. (2011). *Sandtray therapy: A practical manual* (2nd ed.). London: Routledge.

James, W. (1996). *A pluralistic universe*. Lincoln, NB: University of Nebraska Press.

Kennerley, H. (2007). *Socratic method*. Oxford: Oxford Cognitive Therapy Centre, Warneford Hospital.

McLellan, G. (1995). *Pluralism*. Buckingham: Open University Press.

McLeod, J. (2018). *Pluralistic therapy: Distinctive features*. London: Routledge, Taylor & Francis Group.

McLeod, J., & McLeod, J. (2016). Assessment and formulation in pluralistic counselling and psychotherapy. In M. Cooper & W. Dryden (Eds.), *The handbook of pluralistic counselling and psychotherapy*. London: Sage.

Mearns, D., & Thorne, B. (1999). *Person-centred counselling in action* (2nd ed.). In W. Dryden (Ed.). London: Sage.

Merry, T. (2002). Learning and being in person-centred counselling. Ross-onWye: PCCS Books.

Padesky, C. (1993). *Socratic questioning: Changing minds or guiding discovery?* ECBT Keynote address delivered at the European Congress of Behavioural and Cognitive Therapies, London.

Reber, A. R. (1985). *Dictionary of psychology.* England: Penguin Books.

Rogers, C. R. (1957). The necessary and sufficient conditions of therapeutic personality change. *Journal of Consulting Psychology, 21*, 95–103.

Stewart, W. (2013). *An A-Z of counselling theory and practice* (5th ed.). Hampshire: Cengage Learning EMEA.

Twigg, E., & McInnes, B. (2010). *YP-CORE user manual*, Version 1.0, CORE. Rugby: Information Management Systems Ltd.

Verhofstadt-Deneve, L. M. F., Dillen, L., Helskens, D., & Siongers, M. (2004). The psychodramatic "social atom method" with children: A developing dialogical self in dialectic action. In J. J. M. Hermans & G. Dimaggio (Eds.), *The dialogical self in psychotherapy.* Hove: Brunner-Routledge.

Chapter 3

Sand-tray specific mechanisms

It is not the mountain we conquer, but ourselves
(Sir Edmund Hilary, Kuchler, 2003, p. 20)

Hartman and Zimberoff (2009) suggested that the motivation for change comes from an "internal desire for growth" (p. 7). Thus, a client's inner world where change is desired is likely to concern psychological disturbance related to a personal issue.

This intrapsychic experience is a significant feature in sand-tray therapy.

In the pluralistic theoretical framework, the two sand-tray specific mechanisms of phenomenological anchor and phenomenological hook facilitate the counselling process bringing a decrease in psychological and emotional distress.

Objects with significant symbolism are explored at different times during therapy, aided by these mechanisms.

Phenomenological anchor

The phenomenological anchor acts as a point of reference, positioning the beginning of the client's exploration of a particular issue (Fleet, 2019; Fleet et al., 2021). This physical reminder frees the client to engage in "edge of awareness" (Gendlin, 1984) processing. Gendlin (1996) described "the edge" as the "border zone" between the unconscious and the conscious (pp. 17–18). He suggested that when this "edge of awareness" experience emerges, it is a non-verbal felt sense, which Gendlin described as "the implicit". The implicit is vague and fuzzy when it emerges, and Gendlin (1996) was concerned with how creative thinking enabled the implicit in becoming explicit, as the individual finds the right words to express this felt sense.

This point is relevant to sand-tray therapy, which is the ideal context for creative thinking, the symbolic objects facilitating creative expression, making the implicit explicit.

DOI: 10.4324/9781003158707-3

The phenomenological anchor being a physical symbol negates the need to rely on working memory (Baddeley, 1986; Goldstein, 2010) to recall the starting point in the discovery process. Reflective attention has a limited capacity regarding working memory, which needs rehearsal to maintain the thought in mind, which may have a negative impact on discovery (Weissman et al., 2006). This point is particularly pertinent to sand-tray therapy, which incorporates creative discovery and reflection. Besides, Ericsson and Delaney (1999) stated, "working memory capacity (WMC) can hinder creative thinking in the form of insight" (p. 259), reinforcing the significance of the phenomenological anchor assisting creative discovery.

Sometimes a client, who is engaged in talking therapy alone, can lose track of where they began due to ineffective rehearsal in working memory, and this can make the integration of any insight gained problematic. However, the symbolic object in sand-tray therapy is a reference point aiding the process of integration. Pearson and Wilson (2009) argued how integration is an essential process in therapy that is transformational and involves the client making sense of "their experience and start to view their life from a broader perspective" (p. 145).

Furthermore, Goldstein (2010) suggested that fear and anxiety can take up space in working memory, leaving less capacity for cognitive processing. Fear and anxiety are common issues for clients during therapy, and the phenomenological anchor serves as a bridge of return to the starting point of exploration so that any insight gained can be processed and integrated more readily.

Case study: John

John was a man in his late twenties and living alone due to a recent breakdown in his relationship with his fiancée. During the initial assessment, he described himself as feeling numb. John was in shock after his fiancée left him, without giving him any indication, "*Got home and she'd just gone … gone … no word … gone*" (Fleet, 2019, p. 119). He found it difficult to get through the day, becoming more and more withdrawn, describing his situation as him sitting there and staring into space. John felt frozen, felt isolated, and purposely tried to stop himself from crying. In the first session, he placed an object of an owl with blue eyes into the sand (Image 3.1).

He continually touched the owl, lifting it up and down, as he talked:

> *This resembles X, with her for two years. I find it hard nowadays to get emotional and bring it out. I never got the opportunity to say goodbye I have no closure what-so-ever.*
>
> (Fleet, 2019, p. 227; Fleet et al., 2021, p. 10)

John explored the impact of her leaving that way and how hard it was for him to move on, describing how he perceived a change within him, viewing

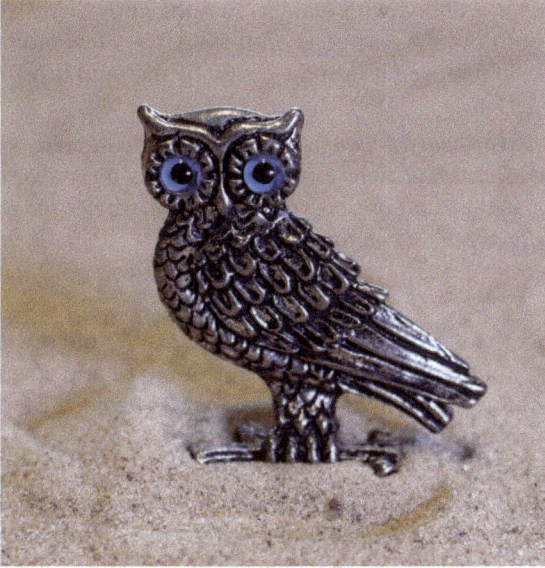

Image 3.1 Owl as a phenomenological anchor representing John's ex-fiancée. (Fleet, 2019, p. 227).

himself as not the same person. The object, acting as a phenomenological anchor, enabled John to explore "edge of awareness" material (Gendlin, 1984). He moved into exploring his perception of how he had lost a part of himself, called his "Cheeky-Chappy," which he symbolised with an object of a comical red devil:

> *Before I was a Cheeky-Chappy, confident … now it doesn't seem like that … I've got issues … I've become vulnerable.*
>
> (Fleet, 2019, p. 228)

John was struggling to engage in life, and the loss he was experiencing had a significant impact on his self-confidence. He expressed a change in his perception of how he was not the same person any more due to the loss of his prized aspect of self (Mearns, 1999; Mearns & Thorne, 2000). Mearns and Thorne described how a person's inner world comprises different parts that have associated feelings and thoughts. They stated, "When walking around inside their existential Self, clients sometimes talk about different "'parts of the Self'" (Mearns & Thorne, 2000, p. 102).

A little further, on in the first session, John touched the owl; "*It's frustrating because I just want to go like that*" (Fleet, 2019, p. 228). As he spoke, he pushed the owl into the sand so it was invisible to the eye. After a few moments of him sitting in silence staring at the spot where the owl was beneath the sand, he began to dig it up, his eyes filled with tears as he spoke how besotted his fiancée was with him, but now she was gone entirely. After a few moments, John reached for the owl and moved it into the centre of the sand tray:

> *I wrote her a letter and although I didn't get nothing back … I feel a weight off my shoulders … after, I had a cry for the first time … a cry that came out of nowhere … and it was all over her … the dog misses her though … that one hurts it really does … I comfort her.*
>
> (Fleet, 2019, p. 229)

As therapy progressed, there was a change in John's attitude, and in session six, he placed the owl in a different position: the bottom left-hand corner of the sand tray. This change in position appeared to represent some distancing or the processing of John's emotion concerning his loss:

> *"Everything is coming really well at the moment,* (picked up the owl) *not really thought about it … I don't feel half as bad".* He continued, *"Sometimes I think … ooh, I haven't thought of X today, but then I think … well, that's a good thing. Her going … it was as good as a death to me because she'd just gone … not a normal break-up … she just dropped off the face of the earth … massive loss … massive."*
>
> (Fleet, 2019, p. 230)

John began to reflect on his experience further:

> *"At one stage last year … the fiancée had left me … I'd lost my job … I was just about to lose my house … but now it is time to move forward and not backwards". "I still love her in a way, but I don't feel like I did … it was horrible … there has been a change … I've become a happier person."*
>
> (Fleet, 2019, p. 230)

He pushed the owl into the sand, so it was invisible to the eye, describing how this had gone further and further into the sand, but this time he left it hidden, without digging it up, buried in the bottom left corner.

The owl, serving as a phenomenological anchor, helped John break new ground to understand the intensity of his loss. He expressed his deep sadness, frustration, and hurt, which had impacted many aspects of his life, including his self-concept. He shared his powerful insight on his loss, *"It was as good as a death to me"* (Fleet, 2019, p. 230). The owl object served as a bridge of return; John integrated his powerful feelings of loss with a new perspective, feeling positive and looking forward to his future. In his words, he *"got closure"* (Fleet, 2019, p. 230).

Phenomenological hook

Gendlin (1996) also argued how material could emerge from the unconscious, originating at such a depth where we cannot sense its source. The concept of phenomenological hook serves as a mechanism, which facilitates unconscious processing (Fleet, 2019; Fleet et al., 2021). The psychodynamic concept of unconscious process (Freud, 1963; Bruschweiler-Stern et al., 2007) is a feature of pluralistic sand-tray therapy. Cooper and McLeod (2011) stated how various methods would "help different people at different points in time ..." (p. 6). They discuss how "CBT can be helpful, *and* person-centred therapy can be helpful, *and* psychodynamic therapy can be helpful ... – in contrast to an 'either/or'" (Castonguay & Beutler, 2006, In Cooper & McLeod, 2011, p. 6) stance.

Besides, the concept of denial is not excluded entirely from person-centred theory as Rogers (1951) stated how overwhelming experiences that "the organism denies to awareness" are not symbolised "into the gestalt of the self-structure" (p. 483–522).

Wilkins (2005) took a PCT stance of mental ill-health and viewed the cause as extreme incongruence.

Similarly, Merry (2002) explained this as an experience that does not fit with the self-concept and results in a person feeling "tense, anxious, frightened or confused" (p. 36).

This process of psychological denial is fundamental to the concept of phenomenological hook, as this mechanism facilitates unconscious processing for the client. The material emerging from the unconscious, previously denied and out of conscious awareness becomes available for processing. In addition, some experience linked to a person's anxiety may be partially symbolised and distorted. Kahn and Rachman (2000) discuss how Rogers described how "Incongruence occurs when experiences in the organism are blocked off from or distorted in self-awareness" (p. 299). For example, the client initially may use a term such as "I am a bit scared," yet later in the therapeutic process can congruently state, "I am terrified," which can then be explored and expressed without denial.

The Jungian perspective of sand-tray work also argues that unconscious processing is a significant feature, with the primary aim for the client to express conflicts, which are still in the unconscious (Turner, 2005). However, the distinction between Jungian sandplay and the pluralistic approach is that in Jungian theory, archetypal symbols used to understand the client's process are not used in the pluralistic approach, as the meaning for each client is unique. The pluralistic therapist who recognises a possible defence in the client will offer an opportunity for the client to work with this, making challenges and suggestions to help explore the material now in conscious awareness.

Jackie created a sand display in session four. She represented two aspects of self by using an ornate egg to represent "*My inner-me*" and an egg with a turtle peeking out of its shell to represent "*My outer-me*". Jackie's "Outer-me" aspect described as the self she shows to the outside world was confident and happy, whilst her "Inner-me" aspect was that anxious part of her she hid from others. Initially, Jackie placed the ornate egg in the centre of the tray and the turtle egg into the top left corner. She touched the turtle egg in the corner and stated, "*I'm kind of keeping a watchful eye ... feeling safe*" (Fleet, 2019, p. 236; Fleet et al., 2021).

This notion of the pluralistic self has been written and discussed by various scholars (Earley & Weiss, 2013; Schmid & Mearns, 2006; Hermans & Dimaggio, 2004; Cooper et al., 2004; Mearns & Thorne, 2000) on their stance on a person having multiple selves, voices, position, configurations, or traces.

Earley and Weiss (2013) identified an aspect of self they named the Inner critic that constantly judges and shames an individual. The self-sabotaging voice of the Inner critic often results in the person feeling inadequate and decreases self-worth. Earley and Weiss expanded this concept and identified seven specific types of Inner critic, including "The Perfectionist, The Inner Controller, The Underminer" (Earley & Weiss, 2013, p. 2), which can threaten the individual's psychological health.

Schmid and Mearns (2006) suggested how "sometimes the difference between the presentational level of the client's self-experiencing and their more fundamental existential self-experiencing is even personified in the form of different parts to the self" (p. 178). The existential aspect being a part of the person's intra-psychic experience – their inner-world.

Hermans and Dimaggio (2004) established a theory of the dialogical self, describing "the self as a multiplicity of parts [voices, characters, positions]" (p. 13). They argued how in dialogical self-theory, the I-position comprised both Internal positions and External positions. The Internal domain consists of alter egos like "I as mother" or "I as singer," and the External extended self, being made up of I-positions such as "my mother," "my husband," or "my enemy." In the External I-position, other people "function in the self as another I" (Hermans & Dimaggio, 2004, p. 20).

Rogers (1951, 1954, 1959) self-theory incorporated various aspects including, the real self (Rogers, 1954), the self-concept, and the ideal self (Rogers, 1951, 1959). Rogers suggested how the real self was "initiated by the actualising tendency, follows organismic valuing, needs and receives positive regard and self regard" (Ahmed & Tekke, 2015, p. 30). Ahmed and Tekke (2015) argued that the real self was the most authentic aspect and part of inner-personality (Ahmed & Tekke, 2015).

The self-concept is understood to be how people perceive themselves, and Rogers argued that a person who grew up in an environment of unconditional positive regard would be psychologically healthy and capable of reaching their full potential as they engage with their actualising tendency (1951, 1959).

However, when a person receives conditional positive regard, any behaviour inconsistent with the conditions of worth is denied or distorted (Rogers,

1961), producing incongruency in the person. Rogers also claimed that a neurotic person is likely to have a self-concept that does not match their experiences and will "distort their experiences to protect themselves or win approval from others" (Aronson et al., 2007, p. 113). Rogers's view of the ideal self is that part of a person who strives to achieve their goals and aspirations (1961), and the closer their self-concept and ideal self is, the more congruent they will be, and experiences truthfully symbolised and the higher their self-worth (1959).

Cooper et al. (2004) aimed to expand Rogers's self-theory and suggested that a person may "develop different self-concepts" (p. 178) due to them experiencing "different kinds of conditional positive regard in...different environments" (p. 178). Cooper et al. (2004) was also interested in "the relationship between the different voices" (p. 178) and that a psychologically healthy individual will have "a dialogical relationship and openness between the different positions" (p. 178). Problems occur when the different parts are objectified within, and there is a disruption to any dialogical relationship.

Mearns and Thorne (2000) theory took a more phenomenological and existential focus when considering self-theory and identified the concept of configurations of self. They described how a configuration made up of innermost feelings and thoughts is associated with their very existence. Mearns (Cooper et al., 2004) also argued that configurations are mostly "incredibly healthy" and "positively adaptive" (p. 180). It is when configurations separate and dissociate that they become problematic (Cooper et al., 2004).

During therapy, it seemed helpful to help Jackie explore both of her aspects of self, and she was invited to move the turtle egg into the centre of the sand tray to bring it more into focus in the session. There was a possibility "*My-Inner-Me*" was split off, or she was experiencing some resistance as Jackie was reluctant to engage with it, placing it in the corner and described this aspect as hiding. Jackie responded to the challenge and moved it next to the ornate egg in the centre, placing a shark object in-between (Image 3.2).

The following discourse occurred:

JACKIE: "*It's a shark ... it's him ... that's me* (surprised tone) *... looking at that, I'm not sure why I have chosen that.*"
DOREEN: "*Okay ... so when you think of a shark ... if you were describing a shark to someone who had never seen or heard of one before what would you say?*" (Socratic Question).
JACKIE: "*Oh ... it's mean ... vicious ... and it attacks ... scary.*"

(Fleet, 2019, p. 235; Fleet et al., 2021, p. 10–11)

Previously, Jackie had tended to move away from her anxious feelings, but at this moment, she stayed with her fear. There was no attempt to minimise this powerful emotion, and she began to express and unpack her fear. As Jackie explored these two aspects of self with the shark sandwiched between,

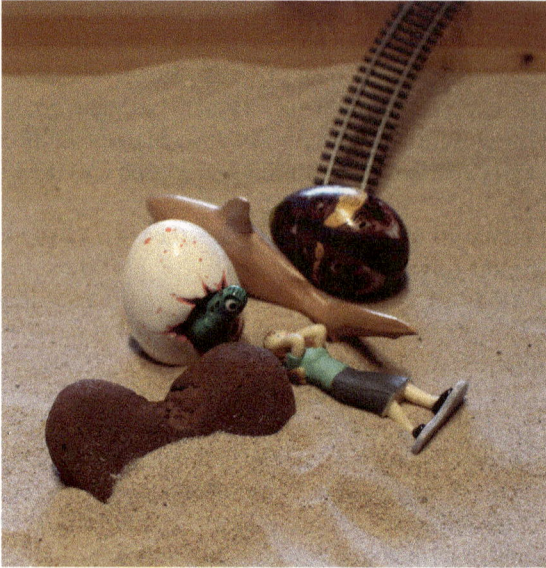

Image 3.2 Jackie's display of her "inner" and "outer" self and the shark object serving as a phenomenological hook helping her explore her fear.
(Fleet, 2019, p. 198).

she began to realise that although she had perceived herself as hiding, staying safe, in reality, she was fearful regarding the threat to her relationship.

Jackie had owned her fear, and in sessions five and six, the turtle egg had gone. By the end of therapy, there appeared to be some integration of these two different aspects of self she called "*My Inner-me*" and "*My outer-me*" as she held the ornate egg in her hand and said, "*This is me … I'm here*". (Fleet, 2019, p. 237).

This process was reiterated in session six when she placed the ornate egg next to the quartz heart representing her partner in the centre of the sand tray again, "*This is me, and this is him*" (Fleet, 2019, p. 237).

Stiles (1997, 1999, 2002b) also talks about a process of integration related to different aspects of self. He identified the "assimilation model" that described how people have different voices, which are experiences that "leave traces and those traces can be reactivated" (Cooper et al., 2004, p. 178). Although most traces are assimilated, some are problematic, and Styles argued that therapy could help "build meaning bridges" (Cooper et al., 2004, p. 178), and by working through those painful voices, integration can occur.

The shark had served as a phenomenological hook to bring Jackie's fear into her conscious awareness for processing. The turtle egg, positioned in the corner of the sand tray representing her hiding from her fear earlier, was moved into the middle and the shark representing her fear placed in-between. This process enabled Jackie to take the observer-experiencer position, resulting in exploring and expressing her previously denied fear. She had built a "meaning bridge" (Stiles, 1999) between her two aspects of self and was no longer denying her fear represented by the removal of the green turtle peeking out of its shell from the sand tray.

In sand-tray therapy, the client can "stay with" their emotional and psychological pain, and various scholars, no matter what their theoretical orientation (Hass-Cohen, 2008; Bradway & McCoard, 1997; Carey, 1999; Kalff, 1980; Plotts et al., 2008; Webber & Mascari, 2008; Woodhouse, 2008), support this claim.

During sand-tray therapy with a client, I have witnessed many times how they do not become overwhelmed but can take the observer-experiencer position (Fleet, 2015). As the experiencer, they also become the observer synonymously; seeing the physical picture in front of their eyes helps them perceive their experience objectively and subjectively (Fleet, 2015). Hawkins (1995) uses the term "experiencer-witness," describing how a client can "step out of their pain" without becoming emotionally distant and can explore their thoughts and feelings, resulting in a reduction in their distress. Malchiodi (2016) suggested how working creatively in this way could help "buffer the hard stuff." As the client takes the dual role of observer-experiencer (Fleet, 2015), establishing a distance between them and their distress enables them to express their painful thoughts and feelings (Malchiodi, 2016).

The combined advantage of the phenomenological anchor and phenomenological hook in pluralistic sand-tray therapy enables both "edge of awareness" discovery and unconscious processing. The symbolic objects placed in the sand facilitate an implicit experience, located at the "border zone" (Gendlin, 1984) to become explicit as the client finds the "right" words to name the experience, and they can gain insight from previously unconscious material processed in conscious awareness.

References

Ahmed, N., & Tekke, M. (2015). Rediscovering Rogers's Self Theory of Personality. *Journal of Educational, Health and Community Psychology, 4*(3), 2088–3129.

Aronson, E., Wilson, T., & Akert, R. (2007). *Social psychology*. New York: Pearson Prentice Hall.

Baddeley, A. D. (1986). *Working memory*. Oxford: Oxford University Press.

Bradway, K., & McCoard, B. (1997). *Sandplay: Silent workshop of the psyche*. New York: Routledge.

Bruschweiler-Stern, N., Lyons-Ruth, K., Morgan, A. C., Nahum, J. P et al. The foundational level of psychodynamic meaning: Implicit process in relation to conflict, defense and the dynamic unconscious. *International Journal of Psychoanalysis*, London *88*, 843–60.

Carey, L. J. (1999). *Sandplay therapy with children and families*. Lanham, MD: Jason Aronson.

Castonguay, L. G., & Beutler, L. E. (2006). Common and unique principles of therapeutic change: What do we know and what do we need to know. In L. G. Castonguary & L. E. Beutler (Eds.), *Principles of therapeutic change that work*. Oxford: Oxford University Press.

Cooper, M., & McLeod, J. (2011). *Pluralistic counselling and psychotherapy*. London: Sage.

Cooper, M., Mearns, D., Stiles W. B., Warner, M., & Elliott, R. (2004). Developing self-pluralistic perspectives and experiential approaches: A round-table dialogue. *Person-Centered and Experiential Psychotherapies, 3*(3), 176–191.

Earley, J., & Weiss, B. (2013). *Freedom from your inner critic: A self-therapy approach*. Colorado: Sounds True Inc.

Ericsson, K. A., & Delaney, P. F. (1999). Long-term working memory as an alternative to capacity models of working memory in everyday skilled performance. In A. Miyake & P. Shah (Eds.), *Models of working memory: Mechanisms of active maintenance and executive control* (pp. 257–291). New York: Cambridge University Press.

Fleet, D. (2015, Spring). Beyond Words: Creative words have an established evidence base when working with children and young people but why are they not more widely used when counselling adults? *Private Practice* (pp. 14–17). British Association for Counselling and Psychotherapy.

Fleet, D. (2019). *Transformation hidden in the sand: Developing a theoretical framework using a sand-tray intervention with adult clients*. Doctoral thesis. Staffordshire University. Stoke-on-Trent. Available from Ethos STORE – Staffordshire Online Repository. https://eprints.staffs.ac.uk/id/eprint/5763

Fleet, D., & Reeves, A., & Burton, A., & DasGupta, M. P. (2021). Transformation Hidden in the Sand: A pluralistic theoretical framework using sand-tray with adult clients. First published online (14 June, 2021). *Journal of Creativity in Mental Health*. https://doi.org/10.1080/15401383.2021.1936738

Freud, S. (1963). *General psychological theory: Papers on metapsychology*. New York: Collier Books-Macmillan Publishing Company.

Gendlin, E. T. (1984). *The client's client: The edge of awareness*. In R. L. Levant & J. M. Shlien (Eds.), *Client-centered therapy and the person-centered approach. New directions in theory, research and practice*. New York: Praeger.

Gendlin, E. T. (1996). *Focusing orientated psychotherapy*. New York: Guildford Press.

Goldstein, E. B. (2010). *Cognitive psychology: Connecting mind, research and everyday experience*. Texas, USA: Wadsworth Publishing.

Hartman, D., & Zimberoff, D. (2009). The hero's journey of self-transformation: Models of higher development from mythology. *Journal of Heart-Centered Therapies, 12*(2), 3–93.

Hass-Cohen, N. (2008). CREATE: Art Therapy Relational Neuroscience Principles (ATR-N). In N. Hass-Cohen & R. Carr (Eds.), *Art therapy and clinical neuroscience*. London: Jessica Kingsley Publishers.

Hawkins, D. R. (1995). *Power VS Force: The Hidden Determinants of Human Behaviour*. London: Hay House.

Hermans, J. J. M., & Dimaggio, G. (2004). *The dialogical self in psychotherapy*. Hove: Brunner-Routledge.

Joseph, S., & Worsley, R. (2005). *Person-centred psychopathology*. Ross-on-Wye, Hertfordshire: PCCS Books.

Kahn, E., & Rachman, A. W. (2000). Carl Rogers and Heinz Kohu: A historical perspective. *Psychoanalytic Psychology, 17*(2), 294–312.

Kalff, D. M. (1980). *Sandplay*. Boston: Sigo Press.

Kalff, D. M. (2003). *Sandplay: A psychotherapeutic approach to the psyche*. Cloverdale, CA: Temenos Press.

Kuchler, B. L. (2003). *That's life: Wit & wisdom*. Minocqua: Willow Creek Books.

Malchiodi, C. A. (2016). Expressive arts therapy and windows of tolerance. *Psychology Today*. Leicester: BPS.

Mearns, D. (1999). Person-centred therapy with configurations of self. *Counselling, 10*(2), 125–130.

Mearns, D., & Thorne, B. (2000). *Person-centred therapy today*. London: Sage Publications Ltd.

Merry, T. (2002). *Learning and being in person-centred counselling* (2nd ed.), Ross-on-Wye: PCCS Books.

Pearson, M., & Wilson, H. (2009). *Using expressive arts to work with mind, body and emotions: Theory and practice*. London: Jessica Kingsley Publishers.

Plotts, C., Lasser, J., & Prater, S. (2008). Exploring sandplay therapy: Application to individuals with traumatic brain injury. *International Journal of Play Therapy, 17*, 138–153.

Rogers, C. R. (1951). *Client-centered therapy: Its current practice, implications and theory*. Boston: Houghton Mifflin.

Rogers, C. R. (1954). *Psycho-therapy and personality change*. Chicago: University of Chicago Press.

Rogers, C. R. (1959). *A theory of therapy, personality and interpersonal relationships, as developed in the client-centered framework*. New York: McGraw-Hill.

Rogers. C. R. (1961). *On becoming a person: A therapist's view of psychotherapy*. Boston: Houghton Mifflin.

Schmid, P. F., & Mearns, D. (2006). Being-with and being-counter: Person-centered psychotherapy as an in-depth co-creative process of personalization. *Person-Centered and Experiential Psychotherapies, 5*(3), 174–190.

Stiles, W. B. (1997). Signs and voices: Joining a conversation in progress. British *Journal of Medical Psychology, 70*, 169–176.

Stiles, W. B. (1999). Signs, voices, meaning bridges, and shared experience: How talking helps. Visiting Scholar Series. Palmerson North, New Zealand: School of Psychology, Massey University.

Stiles, W. B. (2002b). Client-centered therapy with multi-voiced clients: Empathy with whom? In J. C. Watson, R. Goldman, & M. S. Warner (Eds.), *Client-centered and experiential therapy in the 21st century: Advances in theory, research and practice* (pp. 406–414). Ross-on-Wye: PCCS Books.

Turner, B. A. (2005). *The handbook of sandplay therapy*. Cloverdale, CA: Temenos Press.

Webber, J., & Mascari, J. B. (2008). Sand tray therapy and the healing process in trauma and grief counseling. Based on a program presented at the ACA Annual Conference and Exhibition, Honolulu, HI. Retrieved from http://counselingoutfitters.com/vistas/vistas08/Webber.htm

Weissman, D. H., Roberts, K. C., Visscher, K. M., & Woldorff, M. G. (2006). The neural bases of momentary lapses in attention. *Nature Neuroscience, 9*(7), 971–978.

Wilkins, P. (2005). Person-centred theory and "mental illness" In S. Joseph & R. Worsley (Eds.), *Person-centred psychopathology: A positive psychology of mental health* (Chapter 4, pp. 43–59). Hertfordshire: PCCS Books Ltd.

Woodhouse, J. (2008). SANDPLAY: Growing ground in person-centred play therapy. In S. Keys & T. Walshaw (Eds.), *Person-centred work with children and young people: UK practitioner perspectives* (Chapter 4, pp. 29–38). Ross-on-Wye: PCCS Books.

Chapter 4

The dynamic phenomenological field

Courage is resistance to fear, mastery of fear – not absence of fear
(Mark Twain In Klingbell, 2020, p. 12)

It can be a formidable task for a client to begin exploring their inner world, which is likely to consist of conflicting thoughts and fearful feelings, contributing to their emotional and psychological distress. Change can only begin once the person can face, explore, and express such distressing inner experience. Pluralistic sand-tray therapy, using objects representing the client's experience, combined with the collaborative therapeutic relationship, can aid that challenging process so that a phenomenological shift can occur.

The dynamic phenomenological field, within the pluralistic sand-tray framework is defined as:

> The subjective perceptual field of the individual; not static but a dynamic 'space' where the individual strives to understand, perceiving their inner world and external events in their own unique way.
>
> (Fleet, 2019, p. 161)

This field is related to various processes, including phenomenological shift, phenomenological flux, phenomenological distortion/denial, and pre-phenomenological process (Fleet, 2019; Fleet et al., 2021). These processes occur within the person's dialogical intra-psychic experience when engaging in pluralistic sand-tray therapy.

Rogers's (1959) explanation of personality was rooted in the individual's subjective experience, conducive to phenomenological philosophy. Sanders (2006) described how "a phenomenological position is one where we think that the 'truth' about experience is generated within the individual ..." (p. 21), emphasising the point that the truth is subjective and based on the uniqueness of the person.

DOI: 10.4324/9781003158707-4

Phenomenological shift

The concept of phenomenological shift (Fleet 2019; Fleet et al., 2021) is defined as a shift in the client's inner world perceptions of I think, I feel, I believe, I am. This change reduces psychological and emotional distress linked to an issue focused on in therapy.

At the beginning of therapy, Shirley described feeling overwhelmed and trapped by her anxiety, symbolising this by placing an ornate wooden box into the sand with its lid closed, *"Panic came again this week … being in fear, all the time is tiring … I'm boxed in … sometimes I can't breathe"* (Image 4.1; Fleet, 2019, p. 166; Fleet et al, 2021, p. 9).

At this point in Shirley's process, she did not communicate the cause of her anxiety and could only express how she felt emotionally and physically due to her panic. The closed box was a metaphor representing Shirley feeling "boxed in" with the cause not accessible to her at this time; however, as therapy progressed, she gained insight into her fear and was able to bring change, improving her anxiety. In session five, she walked into the counselling room more confidently and took charge immediately. She sat down and began to stab her fingers into the sand, roughing it up, when, for the previous two sessions, she had used small objects (ladder and a small fibrous coconut) to do the same job. The stabbing action took nearly a minute when she began to talk:

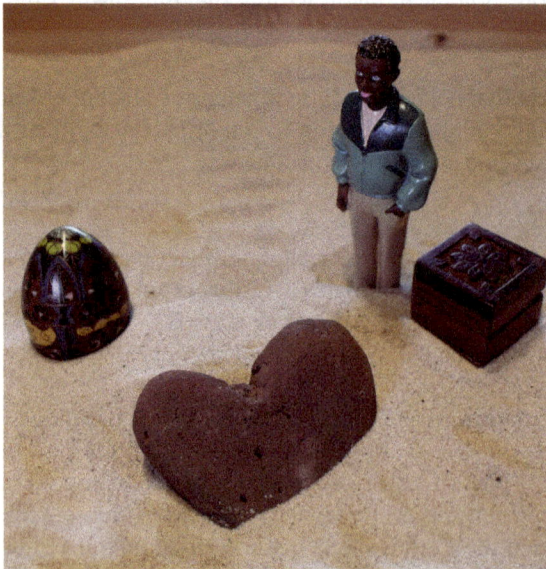

Image 4.1 Shirley feeling trapped by her anxiety symbolised by the closed box.
(Fleet, 2019, p. 165).

SHIRLEY: *"All just a bit too neat"* (roughed up the sand).

DOREEN: *"You're preparing it."*

SHIRLEY: *"Yeah … more natural."*

DOREEN: *"Natural … that feels better for you?"*

SHIRLEY, *"Yeah … don't want it completely flat … need it like … the beach … more natural, the sand is more hilly than before."* (looked sideways for a response).

DOREEN: *"Yeah?"* (Questioning tone).

SHIRLEY: *"Smells like a be … ach … nice sand … last time it didn't have the smell … or is that just me imagining it?"*

DOREEN: *"Don't know, but it was like you could smell it."*

SHIRLEY: *"Mmm."* (Laughed, picked up the ornate wooden box opened it and placed it in the sand).

DOREEN *"You've opened the box!"* (Image 4.2)

SHIRLEY: *"Yeah."*

(Fleet, 2019, pp. 166–169)

Shirley took her time selecting specific objects, then sat back, indicating that she had finished choosing. From a pluralistic perspective, it was essential to acknowledge how Shirley was expressing her agency of roughing up the sand, taking her time to select the objects, then indicated with a glance that she was

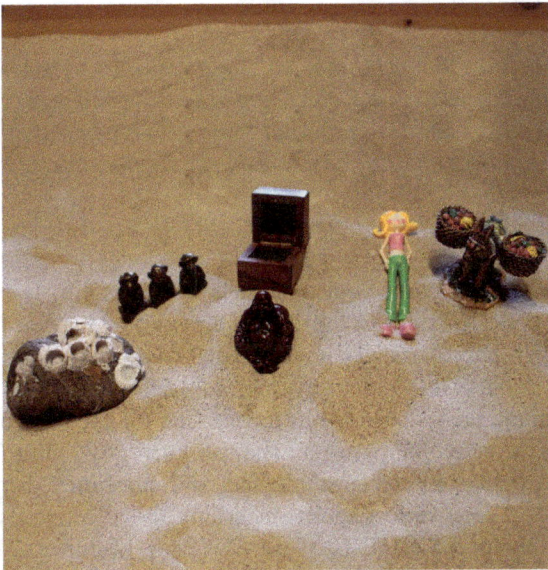

Image 4.2 Shirley experiencing progress symbolised by the open box.
(Fleet, 2019, p. 169).

ready to begin talking. Session five was a breakthrough; opening the lid of the ornate wooden box was significant, and Shirley spoke confidently, *"there is some kind of progress … I'm starting to find new ways to cope with it … not panicking … slowly getting there"* (Fleet, 2019, p. 169; Fleet et al. 2021, p. 9). In a previous session, she explored how fearful she had been about having to leave Africa as a young child (Image 2.3) and move to Britain. Shirley had been happy in Africa but forced to cope in an environment, which was alien and difficult for her, causing much fear. Even as an adult, her perception was that she could be happy and at peace only by returning home to her African roots.

During the sand-tray therapy, Shirley also spoke out loud about the difficult thing she needed to say. This issue involved her questioning her faith, and although she felt pressure to stay faithful to her family's religion, she managed to voice what was inside her head, *"Religion is not real … no … no … not religion … but … but God"* (Fleet, 2019, p. 114). Although this was hard for Shirley to say, she managed to speak the unspoken, and her relief was apparent as her body language became more relaxed.

In the final session, her outlook was different; she felt more positive and placed a large knotted wooden object into the sand next to the Buddha and the open box and described how she was now reaching out like branches and looking forward to new experiences. Furthermore, Shirley was more capable at managing her anxiety by the end of therapy, and there was a shift in her perception of living in Britain, resulting in her feeling happier and more optimistic about her future:

> *It's like a relief … because I thought the only way I can start to feel happy about myself was moving away … but I'm living here at the moment … if I accept that it's not bad … even if it's not what I want, it's not bad at all … I can deal with these problems and still stay here and be comfortable … would be good to be happy here.*
>
> (Fleet, 2019, p. 170)

Shirley had experienced a phenomenological shift in her thoughts, feelings, beliefs, and self-concept. She left therapy more confident and with a new positive outlook, that for her, happiness was now a real possibility. Shirley had unpacked her fear, was coping with her anxiety, and said the "unspoken" and her longing to return home to Africa was put to one side for the time being as she wanted to focus on being happy where she was currently living. This change resulted in a reduction of her psychological and emotional distress, demonstrated by Shirley's positive feedback concerning the effectiveness of therapy, a decrease in her post-CORE-10 score (Twigg & McInnes, 2010), and the final sand display when she constructed a picture representing her new positive outlook.

Phenomenological flux

The concept of phenomenological flux (Fleet, 2019, Fleet et al., 2021) occurs when a client is in conflict, and there is a continuous oscillation between contrasting beliefs, opinions, and feelings. There is no phenomenological shift regarding a specific issue; the client perceives the solution to their problem as external to themselves and outside of their control.

Jackie experienced phenomenological flux regarding her beliefs and feelings concerning whether her partner would stay with her or go back to his wife, whom he was still married to. Jackie's inner conflict was "will he go or will he stay?"

In the first session, she placed a quartz heart in the middle of the sand tray representing her partner and an ornate egg, symbolising her, positioning this next to the heart. Jackie spoke about how she loved going home to be with him at night after work and spending time together. She then placed an object of Pinocchio to represent her partner's wife into the sand:

> *"She's lying to the kids about him...and about me." "I'm trying to enjoy it all but ... waiting for it all to end. When I feel him twitching ... when he goes to see his wife I get a feeling that everything is just going to go ... but it hasn't has it ... I get so stressed over him seeing ... being with her ... he's got an easy route back to her."*
>
> (Fleet, 2019, p. 195)

Here Jackie described the context of her issue and communicated how she was worried that, although she and her partner were happy together, she was concerned he might end up going back to his wife. She moved the quartz heart up and down a piece of rail track with Pinocchio (her partner's wife) at one end and the heart representing her at the other, acting out this threat in a physical way:

> *"You see this is him and that's how it is, he goes down there ... then he is with her and for a little while I feel like this* (picked up an object of a hunched-over figure) *shivering until he comes back."* She walked the crystal back down the track to the ornate egg, *"and I'm like that again* (placed the hunched-over figure in a wooden box) *and that's shut goes back into hiding. He says he's committed but I can't believe it until I see it ... and I have to be super-girl doing all these things ... fun but tiring but if he wasn't there ... erm ... I don't like that idea at all ... he is with me now ... I don't want him to disappear. I feel vulnerable about him ... about her ... feelings of apprehension ... no I don't want to be without him ... absolutely not!"*
>
> (Fleet, 2019, pp. 195–196)

Jackie again began to express her inner-conflict more specifically, moving between feeling secure in her relationship to being apprehensive that her partner may end it and go back to his wife:

> *There's no point in me begging him to stay. His kids might unnerve him, gives me anxiety. We are rock solid ... so together ... I will feel comfortable when I see the divorce paper ... It's very threatening ... I feel in limbo. I kind of block it out.*
>
> (Fleet, 2019, p. 196)

Jackie replaced the train track with a black snake positioning it, with the crystal heart and the ornate egg at on end, and Pinocchio at the other end,

> *There we are ... that is what it looks like at the moment there is the snake, and she keeps pushing it over there to him ... threatening to him.*
>
> (Fleet, 2019, p. 197)

In the following session, Jackie continued to be in flux:

> *"I really don't think he will go home to her ... the connection to her is loosening all the time. He would never go back there ... I feel more certainty."* (Once again she then moved into her fear) *"I'm stuck ... I've not pushed him ... I want to get this going ... we are a unit ... whether he buckles in the end ... thinking ... ooh this isn't worth the trouble ... I feel a threat, lots of ifs and whens."*
>
> (Fleet, 2019, p. 197)

As therapy progressed, Jackie had unpacked her anxiety and fear, but there was still no resolution regarding her perception of the stability of her relationship, and her inner conflict was apparent as she actively worked with the sand tray to explore her turmoil. In the fourth session, Jackie placed an object of a woman with her hands in her hair, laying it down in the centre of the sand tray. She expressed her exasperation concerning her partner, not acting quickly enough to set his divorce in motion.

By session five, Jackie was still in conflict:

> *I'm a little twitchy ... she is the biggest threat to our relationship now ... but he wouldn't just go because she said so. I've always said he'd stay put. But this uncertainty makes me twitchy ... because we are happy at the moment but it might not end up like that.*
>
> (Fleet, 2019, p. 200)

For Jackie, there was no resolution that is apparent in her words, *"it's a scary thing ... he needs to sort it out ... the divorce ... I don't want her* (Pinocchio) *to be a threat ... but she is the biggest threat to our relationship"* (Fleet, 2019, p. 200). She then moved back to reassuring herself once again that he was committing more. However, near the end of this session, she stated:

> I worry whether he thinks he would be better off going back to her ... yeah ... I have a time limit at some point it will be, right I'm done with patience ... not living my life waiting ... need clarity.
>
> (Fleet, 2019, p.200-201)

By the final session, Jackie was still in conflict, *"He hasn't made that move yet ... he's part of my life now ... I'll not push him. He might have to go back if it's too much. I wouldn't like it ... but he might have to go back"* (Fleet, 2019, pp. 200–201). A little further on in this last session, she was still stuck in a state of flux, describing how her partner would prioritise his happiness over any responsibility he had towards his wife, but Jackie worried that things were still not resolved. Her perception of any resolution, she perceived as beyond her control, made any change difficult at this time.

Phenomenological distortion

The concept of phenomenological distortion (Fleet 2019; Fleet et al., 2021) occurs when an experience is distorted and only partially symbolised to manage anxiety related to an overwhelming issue. Humanistic therapy can facilitate the client to become more aware of their organismic experience. Rogers (1980) argued how a client who has experienced favourable conditions in therapy could move "... away from defensiveness towards self-acceptance ..." (p. 440), resulting in "... greater empathy toward their own visceral experiencing" (p. 159). The symbolism of the objects combined with a pluralistic therapeutic relationship offering empathy helps identify distorted phenomenological experience in the client, facilitating them to become more congruent. Rogers stated, "As persons are empathically heard, it becomes possible for them to listen more accurately to the flow of inner experiencing ... thus become more congruent ... more real, more genuine" (1980, pp. 116–117).

In the first three sessions of therapy, Grace began to explore her husband's heavy drinking and the impact this was having on her. She stated:

> *He's like this person ... not evil but this kind of like bad person in a way, in my eyes ... scary ... horrible ... there are good sides to him, but I can't see them ... don't like him when he has had a drink ... I do hope that it won't go on forever, like this ... maybe I can change things.*
>
> (Fleet, 2019, p. 208)

Although Grace expressed some of her difficult feelings concerning her husband's heavy drinking, she still hoped that her husband would change and

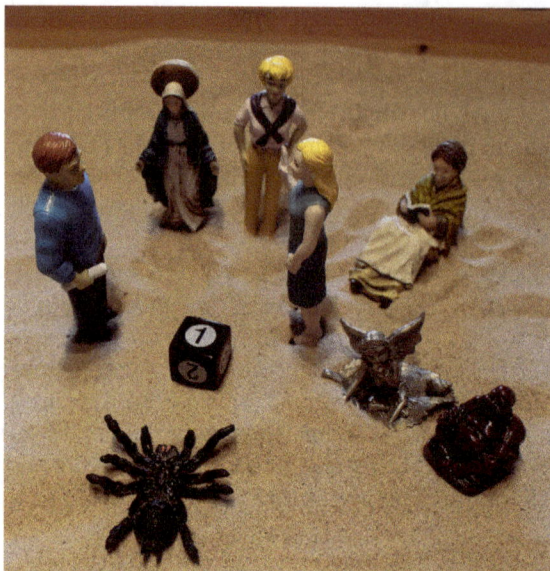

Image 4.3 Grace representing her attempt at some communication with her husband, as
   the full threat to her relationship, is perceived.
(Fleet, 2019, p. 209).

their family would remain intact. In session three, Grace decided to speak to
her husband, aiming to be more transparent about her fears. In the following
session, Grace positioned the objects representing her and her husband facing
each other, then described how she had spoken to him about her concerns and
how he had listened and attempted to reassure her that everything would be
fine. However, later in this session, Grace placed a spider in line with the space
between the objects representing her and her husband (Image 4.3).

The following discourse took place:

GRACE: (Touched the spider) *"It's always there at the back of my mind … so
   this is like this thing … probably … the spider … this thing that … this horrible thing which is always there … at the back of my mind, I suppose even
   though we chatted and stuff."*

DOREEN: *"So this horrible thing which is hidden almost … but you know it is
   there?"*

GRACE: *"Yeah … yeah."*

DOREEN: (tentatively speaks) *"I've … just noticed … you've put the spider
   upside down."*

GRACE: (Laughed) *"Oh yeah (surprised tone) … mmm … yeah maybe …
   maybe it's like trying to hide almost."*

DOREEN: *"Hide?"*

GRACE: *"Yeah ... yeah don't want to kind of confront it ... yeah ... yeah there's a big spider"* (shakes her head).

DOREEN: (Mirrors shake of the head and tentatively speaks) *"So ... when you think of a spider .... on its back ..."*(did not get to ask the complete Socratic question before Grace took the lead).

GRACE: *"It's probably DEAD!"*

DOREEN: *"Dead?"*

GRACE: *"Suppose ... like the end of the relationship ... is the relationship DEAD!"*

(Fleet, 2019, p. 210; Fleet et al., 2021, p. 13)

Grace sat quietly and stared at the sand tray for a while before speaking:

> *And it's right between us ... I don't think he had ever thought ... he just dismissed it ... oh god ... we could just end up splitting up ... it's awful ... but it's just hopeless ... the spider it's between us he doesn't see it ... we could definitely end up splitting up ... dead spider ... like the end of the relationship.*

(Fleet, 2019, p. 211)

The symbolic object of the spider, along with the partly asked Socratic question, had helped Grace realise the threat to her relationship. There was surprise in her voice as she acknowledged that the end of her relationship was a real possibility.

In the following session, Grace used the spider again but placing it the right way up. The spider was in line with the objects representing her and her husband again, but they were further apart (Image 4.4); she described how her husband was still drinking and noticed how the object representing her had its hand up as if saying goodbye to him.

Grace began to congruently explore how the impact her husband's heavy drinking was having on their relationship and her:

> *"I just need to let go ... he's dragging me down". "That scary object is still there ... creeping towards us ... it was on its back last time ... now something bad or scary could be getting closer ... yeah ... his drinking coming forward."*

(Fleet, 2019, p. 212)

Phenomenological denial

The concept of phenomenological denial (Fleet, 2019; Fleet et al., 2021) occurs when unconscious material, which is out of awareness, is not symbolised and an experience that is overwhelming to the individual is

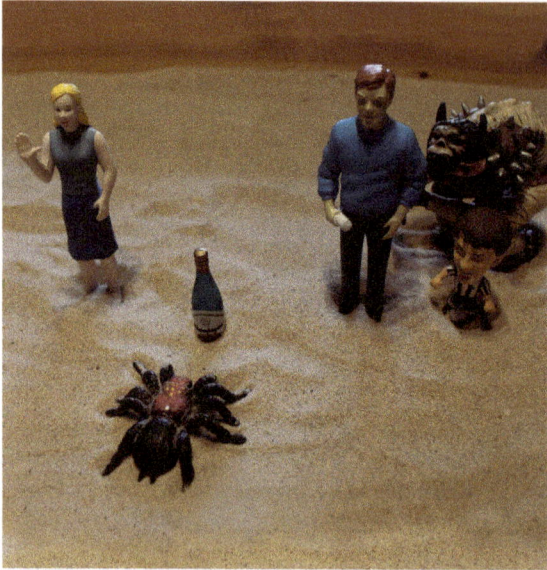

Image 4.4 Grace and the spider "moving towards them" symbolising the probability of her relationship ending.

(Fleet, 2019, p. 212).

denied. The client and the therapist can work with the symbolic objects that aid unconscious processing, with the material moving into consciousness for processing.

Case study: Ruth

As a young child, Ruth shouldered the responsibility of caring for her younger siblings. She had experienced psychological and physical abuse by her mother and was not allowed to engage in the usual fun things that her brothers and sisters did. In the second session, Ruth placed three objects of tiny babies into the sand (Image 4.5).

Ruth stared at the objects of three tiny babies and in a surprised tone said:

RUTH: *"I don't know why I chose them … don't know why I'm looking at these?"*

DOREEN: "No?"

RUTH: *"I don't know why? … I don't know why?"* (pauses).
   "OH (surprised tone) *… if anybody has a baby I'm going to die … oh, I don't want to be a Nana!"* (Fleet et al., 2021, p. 13)

DOREEN: *"You don't?"*

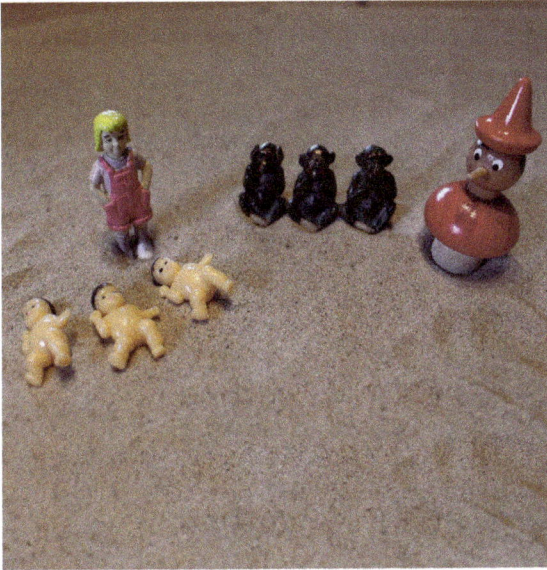

Image 4.5 Ruth demonstrating unconscious processing.
(Fleet, 2019, p. 220).

RUTH: *"No … no … no … I'm too young … it'll be can you look after them … I would want to see them but I don't want to be looking after them … would be stuck."*

DOREEN: *"So you want to hold on to your freedom?"*

RUTH: *"If my kids have kids … they'll trap me … hate the sound of the word Nana … I hate the sound.*
I'd hate it … I'd be trapped … I'd be stuck with their kids, I'd feel old." (Fleet et al., 2021, p. 14)

DOREEN: *"Feeling trapped … and feeling old … hate the thought of it."*

RUTH: *"Yeah … I do … been there done that … now I can go wherever I want. I'm a bit of a gipsy really."* (Fleet et al., 2021, p. 14).

DOREEN: *"Free to be you."*

RUTH: *"Definitely … can't give that up now."* (Fleet et al., 2021, p. 14).

(Fleet, 2019, p. 220)

Ruth's unconscious experience of hating the thought of becoming a Nana, symbolised by the objects of three babies and now being manifested in a physical picture, was available for processing. As she engaged with the therapy, the previously unconscious material was now available for processing, and her strong feelings of not wanting to become a "Nana" emerged. She expressed surprise in terms of what the objects (phenomenological hook) symbolised and explored her powerful feeling of wanting to be free, which she valued as a part of her self-concept. Ruth communicated the intensity of her feelings if she became a Nana when she expressed that she would die if any of her children had a baby. There could be no compromise for Ruth as she gave a high value to her configuration of self (Mearns, 1999): the "gipsy" in her. In later sessions, Ruth began to explore her need for freedom, and she planned "moving away" as part of her future despite the prospect of her family expanding. Ruth's experience was "transferred from the inner world to the outer world and made visible" (Kalff, 2003), facilitating the implicit in becoming explicit as she was able to vocalise her dread of becoming a Nana.

Pre-phenomenological process

> Pre-phenomenological process is described as the participant 'setting the scene', using descriptive communication relating to the context of an issue. This concept is viewed as a precursor for some participants prior to engaging in their phenomenological process.
>
> (Fleet, 2019, p. 221; Fleet et al., 2021)

This essential step for some clients can help them describe enough context before engaging in more profound discovery, and at this time, the therapist required to be a respectful and empathic listener offers the client sufficient space to communicate the facts of their story.

Shirley began talking about her experience of beginning school in Europe after leaving Africa, and there was a need to set the context before she moved into exploring her phenomenological experience:

SHIRLEY: *"My English improved so it was okay … then about year eight, they decided to move me because I was a year older. So in year eight, I met all my friends and everything and then they moved me to year ten."* (Fleet, 2019, p. 222).

Shirley went on to describe more about the school she was in and the class she was moved to before she was ready to explore in a deeper way:

SHIRLEY: *"That is when I realized that it actually started."*
DOREEN: *"It?"*
SHIRLEY: *"The anxiety."*
DOREEN: *"So you were moved up because you were a year older and you lost your friends?"*

(Fleet, 2019, p. 222)

By setting the scene, Shirley was then able to explore her phenomenological experience of loss and her perception of when her anxiety began.

SHIRLEY: *"Yeah ... it kind of changed everything because I lost all ... I felt like I lost them ... not seeing them as much ... and being thrown into an entirely different group ... we were all the same age but I felt younger because I was in the year below before ... it was always weird."*

DOREEN: *"Weird?"*

SHIRLEY: *"Yeah and my mum said it wasn't that bad ... but it IS a big deal ... I came home and I was panicking!"*

(Fleet, 2019, p. 222)

Shirley began to explore how frightening this change was for her, making her feel so different from the rest of the group and her perception of her experience being weird and an outsider was a theme that continued into her adult years.

Another example of pre-phenomenological process occurred partway through Anne's first session. She began talking about herself as a young woman who left home and moved to a big city:

I went to live in X for three years ... served in the bars as a barmaid and I used to work ten till three then half five until eleven, and we'd have a lock-in, and I'd go to all-night parties .... mmm. I always kept active ... very disciplined.

(Fleet, 2019, p. 222)

Anne continued to describe for a few minutes how active she was in the past before I offered a reflection:

DOREEN: *"So you were very active in the past."*

ANNE: *"And not just when I was younger ... but now,* (became tearful) *I can't accept it* (cries) *even going upstairs hurts."*

DOREEN: *"Almost like this isn't me ... it can't be ..."*

ANNE: *"Yeah ... I've lost who I am"* (continued to cry).

(Fleet, 2019, p. 223)

Setting the scene was necessary so that Anne could be understood, and I, as listener, would not need to ask factual finding questions. Any questions at this time would have interrupted her flow. Then, when there was a pause, the reflecting statement of being very active in the past helped her to begin expressing her thoughts and feelings related to her loss.

References

Fleet, D. (2019). *Transformation hidden in the sand: Developing a theoretical framework using a sand-tray intervention with adult clients.* Doctoral thesis. Staffordshire University. Stoke-on-Trent. Available from Ethos STORE – Staffordshire Online Repository. https://eprints.staffs.ac.uk/id/eprint/5763

Fleet, D., & Reeves, A., & Burton, A., & DasGupta, M. P. (2021). Transformation hidden in the sand: A pluralistic theoretical framework using sand-tray with adult clients. First published online (14 June, 2021). *Journal of Creativity in Mental Health*. https://doi.org/10.1080/15401383.2021.1936738

Kalff, D. (2003). *Sandplay: A psychotherapeutic approach to the psyche*. Cloverdale, CA: Temenos Press.

Mearns, D. (1999). Person-centred therapy with configurations of self. *Counselling*, *10*(2), 125–130.

Rogers, C. R. (1959). A theory of therapy, personality and interpersonal relationships, as developed in the client-centered framework. In S. Koch (Ed.), *Psychology: A study of science. Vol. 3: Formulations of the person and the social context* (pp. 184–256). New York: McGraw-Hill.

Rogers, C. R. (1980). *A way of being*. Boston, New York: Houghton Mifflin Company.

Sanders, P. (2006). *The person-centred counselling primer: A concise, accessible, comprehensive introduction*. Ross-on-Wye: PCCS Books.

Twain, M. (1894). Pudd'nhead Wilson in *The Century Magazine, 47*(5),772. In G. A. Klingbell (2020), This one fear. *Faculty Publications*. 3154. https://digitalcommons.andrews.edu/pubs/3154

Twigg, E., & McInnes, B. (2010). *YP-CORE user manual*, Version 1.0, CORE. Rugby: Information Management Systems Ltd.

Chapter 5

Additional benefits characteristic of sand-tray therapy

The real voyage of discovery consists not in seeking new lands but seeing with new eyes

(Marcel Proust, 1908. www.age-of-the-sage.org/)

Therapists who had never considered using sand tray may be unaware of the specific advantages particularly relevant to this approach. When aware of the benefits, a therapist might decide to incorporate sand tray into their practice and help the client gain from the advantages concerning the processes of:

- Touch
- The spatial arrangement of objects
- Moving and removing objects
- Burying objects and manipulating the sand

These elements contribute to the therapeutic process in a specific way for each client, enhancing the therapeutic process and easing the client's emotional and psychological distress (Fleet, 2019; Fleet et al., 2021).

Touch

Touch is a topic written by scholars from various disciplines, including counselling (Wright, 2020; Moy, 1981), psychotherapy (Phelan, 2009; Smith et al., 1998), social work (McKinney & Kempson, 2012; Strozier et al., 2010), and nursing (Kelly et al., 2017; Routasala, 2001). Often, quotes on touch have an emotive quality, emphasising its importance in human experience. Montague stated, "Touch is the mother of all senses" (1971, p. 3) and described how "both truth and communication begin with a simple gesture: touch, the authentic voice of feeling." (1971, p. 287).

The vast majority of the literature on touch focuses on therapist–client touch, exploring the pros and cons of this behaviour in therapy. Boundary-crossing can occur when a client may misinterpret a therapist's touch, and

DOI: 10.4324/9781003158707-5

Alyn (1988) suggested that this could involve the "risk of obscuring the line between erotic and non-erotic touch" (p. 432). In 1972, Wolberg was more definitive in his stance on touch in psychotherapy and argued how "physical contact with the patient is absolutely a taboo (since it may) mobilize sexual feelings in the patient and the therapist" (p. 606).

Conversely, in some humanistic therapies, non-erotic touch is viewed as behaviour that can enhance the therapeutic relationship and facilitate the counselling process (Williams, 1997; Holroyd & Brodsky, 1977).

However, if a client did misconstrue a therapist's intentions regarding touch, the therapist would need to address this using immediacy, helping the client clearly understand the motivation behind the therapeutic touch. A therapist uses the skill of immediacy to help a client work "in the 'here and now', within the dynamic of the counsellor-client relationship" (Milne, 2003, p. 46). Such immediacy is an ethical requirement in order to set safe boundaries for both client and therapist.

Although touch between therapist and client in sand-tray work has the same benefits and pitfalls, boundary-crossing is a risk that does not apply to the client when touching the sand and objects. This additional dimension of touch provides benefits discussed in greater detail in the following paragraphs.

During sand-tray therapy, clients can pinch the grains of sand between fingers and thumb, use their fingers in a stabbing action to rough up the sand, and sometimes smooth it flat. Markell (2002) argued how this type of behaviour is a dialogue between the internal and the external world, a blend between the psyche and the physical.

The client constructs a physical picture in the sand using the symbolic objects to represent their inner experience. In contrast to Lambert's (1991) warning of how touch between therapist–client can harm the therapeutic alliance, touching the sand and objects in sand-tray therapy can empower the client, positively impacting the therapeutic relationship. Turner (2005) highlighted how such intentional manipulation of the sand conveys client autonomy and emotional release.

Turner's view was that this type of touch is a mirror to the Self, and in the presence of an accepting therapist, it "establishes relationship of Self to other" (2005, p. 211). Physical touch helps the emotion be expressed and processed, and Turner (2005) suggested how the act of physically pushing an object into the sand might be interpreted as an expression of the client's autonomy. Additionally, a specific emotion such as anger might be linked to this action.

Homeyer and Sweeney (2011) described how anxious clients who handle the objects become relaxed and more readily engaged. Moreover, when clients let the sand sift through their fingers, they find this action self-soothing, which helps them to begin talking, "It's almost as if the touching of the sand facilitated the loosening of the tongue" (Homeyer & Sweeney, 2011, p. 32). Turner (2005) identified certain emotions with the type of touch and suggested how a client digging in the sand could express their anger, whilst smoothing the sand could represent feelings of tenderness. Montague (1971) argued how "touch is a language of its own with a large vocabulary" (p. 314) and extended this concept by suggesting, "through touch, we communicate what cannot be spoken, for touch is the true voice of feeling" (Montague, 1971, p. 314). Furthermore, Montague argued how synonymous touch and feeling are and stated, "Emotion, feeling, affect and touch are scarcely separable from one another" (1971, p. 288).

Further evidence of the benefit of touch in sand-tray therapy comes from neurobiological literature. Badenoch (2008) suggested how sand-tray therapy stimulates the regulation of right-brain processes and argued how this could facilitate the processing of painful and dissociated experiences. Mild dissociation can involve a mild emotional detachment from the immediate environment (Dell, 2006), sometimes described as a coping mechanism to minimise stress, boredom, or conflict (Weiten & Lloyd, 2008). Pathological dissociation can be a dissociative disorder, possibly triggered by trauma (Abugel & Simeon, 2006). Such severe dissociation can include loss of memory, a sense of self that seems unreal, and being diagnosed with multiple personality disorder (Abugel & Simeon, 2006).

Ammann (1991) supported the argument that right-brain processes helped access emotional experience and described how the right hemisphere works with non-verbal images, playing a significant role in emotional expression. Once the client touches the sand, the hypothesis is that integration commences due to an instant connection between body emotion and thought (Badenoch, 2008).

Badenoch's (2008) understanding of this process is described as the sensation of touching the sand, proceeds from the fingers up to the thalamus, then to the parietal lobe in the brain, associated with touch. Then as the therapist offers empathy, the client can explore their painful experience, "new synapses carry that information throughout the brain, and blood flow changes course to more soothing paths" (Badenoch, 2008, p. 12).

More contemporary research (De Little, 2020) supports the link between biology and emotional regulation, arguing how neuroscientific research has furthered understanding of how using the sand tray can be a powerfully transformative experience for clients.

Sometimes, a client may be reluctant to touch the sand, and the therapist needs to avoid assuming why this is. There will be a reason why a client will demonstrate avoidance, and any therapeutic intervention aimed at exploring this will depend on the therapist's theoretical orientation. Turner (2005) saw untouched sand as most likely related to a difficulty or block that needed to be worked on, which relates to unconscious fears.

However, Turner (2005) was still tentative in her interpretations of untouched sand by a client and warned therapists to avoid making assumptions, as each client will have their unique reason for any reluctance.

In humanistic therapy, reluctance to touch the sand or engage in the sand-tray process could be interpreted as the client experiencing a state of "edge of awareness" (Gendlin, 1996). Clients who cannot find the "right" words to describe their experience may exhibit "stuckness," having an implicit know-ingness but cannot explicitly communicate this. The symbolic objects used by the client, along with the therapist's interventions, may help overcome this block. The client may begin to touch the sand, and the object/s and the symbolism can help in guided discovery, involving cognitive and emotional processes. Often, clients will gain insight resulting in them finding the "right" words to communicate their experience. However, a safe environment and a trusting therapeutic relationship are essential for the guided discovery process, so the client feels comfortable enough to trust and become engaged.

Hass-Cohen (2008) also argued that working creatively in therapy using sensory experiences of touch and vision contributes to processing emotions and facilitates therapeutic change. Montague (1986) describes how sometimes a visual experience feels inadequate, and "touch adds the missing dimension and completes the experience" (p. 311).

Furthermore, Badenoch (2008) suggested how clients would experience a release of tension when they touch the sand or objects. If the therapist were to reflect on this action, it might help the client connect physically in the "here and now" in the sand-tray session. An example of such a reflection is, "as you hold that object very softly in your hands and speak, you appear more relaxed." Here, the therapist reflects the client's body language as they speak, which may help them become more engaged and explore deeper.

All the clients in the case study research touched the sand and objects at different times. Some roughed up the sand, such as Shirley, who described her action to make it look and feel more natural, more like a beach. The beach-like link of roughing up the sand helped Shirley talk about a vivid and treasured memory of the beach in Africa when she was a child, and she talked for some time about her wonderful experience back then. Therapists need to stay alongside the client in their experiencing and value good and positive experiences as well as helping clients to talk about their pain and distress.

Jackie touched the objects in every session, moving them about, projecting her thoughts and feeling onto them. For Jackie, touch was an integral part of her therapeutic process. Likewise, John was very active with both the sand and the objects and continually pinched the sand grains together at times and held various objects in his hands as he spoke and expressed his feelings. The significant objects acted as phenomenological anchors for Jackie and John, positioned the beginning of their exploration linked to a specific issue.

This representation had the effect of freeing them to explore "edge of awareness" experience (Gendlin, 1984) at various times, where they both went further in their discovery and gained insight (Fleet, 2019).

Spatial arrangement of the objects

In sand-tray therapy, the spatial arrangement of the objects is important to the therapeutic process. Often, significant objects are placed in the centre of the sand tray, helping the client focus on a particular issue. Turner (2005) viewed the centre of the sand tray as a central element to the client's progression.

In the case study, Ruth placed an object of a demon monster into the centre of the sand tray in the first session and immediately began to explore the psychological and physical abuse she had experienced by her mother. This symbolic object brought up powerful feelings for her, and she stated, "*That reminds me of my mum ... she was always vile to me when I was growing up ... she'd say horrible things to me ... and hit me with a cane*" (Fleet, 2019, p. 130). Ruth explained how she had worked on this issue by talking to trusted friends but needed to revisit it first before talking about anything else. She almost entirely focused on her abuse throughout the first session and introduced her problem of being unable to form a romantic relationship with a man only near the end of this session. In the remainder of the sessions, she focused on other issues, including her self-concept and problems she had experienced with her friends.

Near the end of her therapy, Ruth placed an object of a female holding a walking frame into the centre of the sand and stated, "*She's like a little frail old lady ... she wants to go home ... brings tears to my eyes*" (Fleet, 2019, p. 187; Fleet et al., 2021, p. 12). This object, acting as a phenomenological anchor that represented her mother, who was now in a nursing home, helped Ruth explore further, and her perception of her mother began to shift. There was a change in Ruth's view of her mother being an abusive figure to her now being vulnerable. Ruth expressed her sympathy but also her freedom, "*... it happened, and I can't do anything about it because it's already in the past, and I can do anything I want now, can't I?*" (Fleet, 2019, p. 188).

Turner (2005) suggested that objects representing issues worked through in earlier sessions are often brought to the centre later on during the process of integration. Another object can also replace the significant object representing progress and placed in the centre (Fleet, 2019). In her end-of-therapy feedback, Ruth indicated her progression, "*Took a look into what my feelings from the past mean ... I'm getting to grips with them*" (Fleet, 2019, p. 246).

In addition, the corners of the sand tray also appear to have a significant part to play in the therapeutic process. Sometimes, an object will be placed in a corner that may relate to a client attempting to avoid an experience, which is fearful. This behaviour might be a conscious decision with the client stating, "I'm not going to talk about that today' or an unconscious act linked to a defence".

Jackie placed the object of a small turtle peeking out of its shell in the top right-hand corner of the sand tray (Chapter 3). She described how this represented her staying safe and hiding away from the conflict concerning her partner's estranged wife. However, as therapy progressed, Jackie realised that she could not stay safe but was fearful that her relationship might end. This insight emerged once Jackie accepted the invitation to position the object in the centre of the sand tray when she began to acknowledge and work through her fear.

John also used the corners in his sand-tray work. At the beginning of therapy, he placed the owl representing his ex-fiancée, who had left him in the centre.

However, at the end of therapy, he placed the owl in the bottom left corner symbolising how he would never forget her but now had closure and could move on. He demonstrated his sense of closure further by pushing the owl beneath the sand, still positioned in the corner, stating, "*and she's gone further and further into the sand*" (Fleet, 2019, p. 230).

Moving an object around the sand tray

Moving the objects around the sand tray is a common occurrence in sand-tray therapy, enabling a client to bring their emotions and experience into the "here and now." Homeyer and Sweeney (2011) argued how the sand tray is a projective medium that facilitates the processing of intra- and interpersonal experience, with the client able to act out difficult or fearful emotions. Kalff (2003) suggested that projecting onto the objects gives a therapeutic distance for clients who can safely express their emotions. They can adopt the observer-experiencer position, enabling them to take one step out of their pain but remain connected to the experience (Fleet, 2015).

Jackie consistently moved the objects around the sand tray, bringing her experience, causing her anxiety into the "here and now." She used a ladder placed on the outside edge of the tray, symbolising and acting out her desire for escape, a piece of rail-track for moving objects up and down to represent a threat to her relationship and placed objects representing negative relationships further away from the objects symbolising her.

Adding an object to the sand tray

During sand-tray therapy, the use of objects is an active and ongoing process with the client as the main driver behind the work.

Most clients will construct an initial picture in the sand but will often add objects as the session progresses. Every action, including the search for a particular object, may be significant to their process. Even when a client cannot find the ideal object they are searching for, a flexible choice to make another fit with their symbolism can be an empowering experience. It can help if the therapist prizes the client's creativity and adaptability by commenting, "Aah, you made it fit!" This response viewed as respecting the client as it acknowledges their input.

However, Rogers used the term "prizing," which "communicated a greater intensity of feeling" (Mearns & Thorne, 1998, p. 66) and involved valuing the client unconditionally.

Furthermore, therapists need to avoid apologising for not having the ideal object and acknowledge the one chosen by the client even when it may be a stone, shell, or something far removed from the initial target object. Once the client begins to explore the symbolism, the object will take on the meaning assigned to it by the client.

Removing an object from the sand tray

A client may physically remove an object from the sand tray and have a particular reason for this. The motivation may be that the object has a powerful and emotive symbolism that is overwhelming for the client at that time, and they want to remove it due to them not being ready to acknowledge their pain. Alternatively, this action might represent the desire for change, and they want someone or something gone from their life, and the autonomous removal of the object can be a symbol for that desire. Whatever the reason, a purposeful discussion on this action can be helpful to the client's process.

Case study: Anne

Anne began her first session by placing an object of a woman sitting in a wheelchair in the centre of the sand. She spoke through her tears as she expressed her fear that she would not completely recover and would be left unable to walk due to her severe accident. Anne reached out and took the object out of the sand tray, turning it around, facing it away from her, saying, "*I don't want to look at her*" (Fleet, 2019, p. 177). The object and its removal had a cathartic (Thurschwell, 2009) effect on Anne, and she broke down and sobbed. Once her sobbing had subsided, Anne was asked whether she was okay to carry on, wanted to stop, or needed a break. Anne replied that she did want to carry on but had not cried about it before. Even though her tears had been bubbling near the surface, she had continued to push them down until today.

Berndtson (1975) described how catharsis involves powerful expression that can bring change and freedom of emotion. Bandes (2009) also views catharsis as a helpful process in therapy that can give the client closure due to the release of emotions associated with an unresolved issue. Nevertheless, there is disagreement amongst some theorists on how helpful catharsis is. Markman et al. (1993) focused on the cathartic expression of anger and suggested how some people can feel angrier than before the catharsis process. However, other scholars (Reeck et al., 2016; Frattaroli, 2006) view catharsis as therapeutic.

In sand-tray therapy, the process of externalising and projecting onto the objects in a physical space with definite boundaries facilitates a client to stay with their pain and not become overwhelmed. For Anne, she had control over removing the object that symbolised her pain and, after expressing her fear, could continue with the remainder of the session.

Burying objects in the sand

It is pretty common for clients to bury objects into the sand during therapy. Depending on the client and the issue explored, there will be different reasons for this. John demonstrated his frustration by pushing the owl object representing his ex-fiancée who had left him into the sand (Fleet, 2019, p. 120). After digging it up, he expressed how he felt stuck in his grief and could not make any sense why his fiancée had left him without her offering any reason for ending their relationship (Chapter 5). The digging up of the owl represented John's intention to explore his loss rather than leave it buried. Turner (2005) would appear to support this understanding and argued, "burying and then digging up may indicate a new capacity to face things that were once overpowering" (p. 307).

In session two, John placed the owl in the sand again and placed an object of a pig next to it, saying, "*What I love*". He then held the pig in his hand, saying, "*My dog ... she's going to be okay*", and then buried it up to its neck in the sand, stating (Image 5.1), "*She's not going anywhere*" (Fleet, 2019, p. 229).

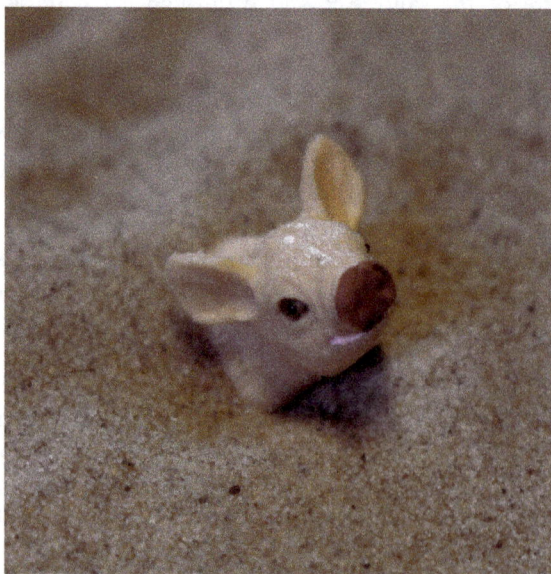

Image 5.1 John symbolising the love he still had.
(Fleet, 2019, p. 229).

In this part of his process, John was exploring the love he had lost, relating to his fiancée, "*Just can't move on until she's gone … out of my mind*" (Fleet, 2019, p. 229), and the love he still had with his dog. He had used the action of burying significant objects that held different meanings for him: the owl represented the love he had lost, and the pig represented the love he still had.

The protective object

Sometimes, a client can appear stuck in their fear, which can block any progress. A fearful object such as a monster often represents the client's fear, and it can be difficult for the client to explore their experience when their attention is focused entirely on the threatening object. It can help the client if the therapist suggests selecting a protective object to help shift their focus. An example of a therapeutic intervention is 'It seems that the monster has much power … I'm wondering if you could have a protective object which you could place in the sand; what would that be?' Clients often respond to this suggestion by selecting a protective object that might have a spiritual or a religious connotation, such as an angel or the Buddha or the Virgin Mary. Others might select a power animal such as a lion or a tiger. The protective object is usually placed close to the threatening one, giving a sense of diminishing the power of the threat.

References

Abugel, J., & Simeon, D. (2006). *Feeling unreal: Depersonalization disorder and the loss of self*. Oxford: Oxford University Press.

Alyn, J. (1988). The politics of touch in therapy: A response to Willison and Masson. *Journal of Counseling and Development, 66*, 432–433. https://doi.org/10.1002/j.1556-6676.1988.tb00906.x

Ammann, R. (1991). *Healing and transformation in sandplay*. LaSalle, IL: Open Court.

Badenoch, B. (2008). *Being a brain-wise therapist: A practical guide to interpersonal neurobiology*. London: W. W. Norton.

Bandes, S. A. (2009). Victims, 'closure', and the sociology of emotion. *Law and Contemporary Problems, 72*(2), 1–26. Retrieved from http://scholarship.law.duke.edu/lcp/vol72/iss/2/2/

Berndtson, A. (1975). *Art, expression and beauty*. Florida, United States: Krieger.

De Little, M. M. (2020). Using the sand tray in the context of the latest research in neuroscience to transform clients' defences. *Canadian Journal of Counselling and Psychotherapy, 54*(3), 259–285.

Dell, P. F. (2006). A new model of dissociation identity disorder. *The Psychiatric Clinics of North America, 29*(1), 1–26, vii.

Fleet, D. (2015, Spring). Beyond Words: Creative words have an established evidence base when working with children and young people but why are they not more widely used when counselling adults? *Private Practice* (pp. 14–17). British Association for Counselling and Psychotherapy.

Fleet, D. (2019). *Transformation hidden in the sand: Developing a theoretical framework using a sand-tray intervention with adult clients.* Doctoral thesis. Staffordshire University. Stoke-on-Trent. Available from Ethos STORE – Staffordshire Online Repository. https://eprints.staffs.ac.uk/id/eprint/5763

Fleet, D., & Reeves, A., & Burton, A., & DasGupta, M. P. (2021). Transformation hidden in the sand: A pluralistic theoretical framework using sand-tray with adult clients. First published online (14 June, 2021). *Journal of Creativity in Mental Health.* https://doi.org/10.1080/15401383.2021.1936738

Frattaroli, J. (2006). Experimental disclosure and its moderators: A meta-analysis. *Psychological Bulletin, 132*(6), 823–865.

Gendlin, E. T. (1984). *The client's client: the edge of awareness.* In R. L. Levant and J. M. Shlien (Eds.). Client-centered therapy and the person-centered approach. New directions in theory, research and practice. New York: Praeger.

Gendlin, E. T. (1996). *Focusing orientated psychotherapy.* New York: Guildford Press.

Hass-Cohen, N. (2008). CREATE: Art therapy relational neuroscience principles (ATR-N). In N. Hass-Cohen & R. Carr (Eds.), *Art therapy and clinical neuroscience.* London: Jessica Kingsley Publishers.

Holroyd, J. C., & Brodsky, A. M. (1977). Psychologists' attitudes and practices regarding erotic and nonerotic physical contact with patients. *American Psychologist, 32*, 843–849. https://doi.org/10.1037/0003-066X.32.10.843

Homeyer, L. E., & Sweeney, D. S. (2011). *Sandtray therapy: A practical manual* (2nd ed.). London: Routledge.

Kalff, D. (2003). *Sandplay: A psychotherapeutic approach to the psyche.* Cloverdale, CA: Temenos Press.

Kelly, M. A., Nixon, L., McClurg, C., Scherpbier, A., King, N., & Dornan, T. (2017). Experience of touch in healthcare: A meta-ethnography across the healthcare professions. *Qualitative Health Research*, 1–13. https://doi.org/10.1177/1049732317707726

Lambert, M. J. (1991). *Introduction to psychotherapy research.* In L. E. Beutler & M. Cargo (Eds.), *Psychotherapy research: An international review of programmatic studies* (pp. 1–11). Washington, DC: American Psychological Association.

Markell, M. J. (2002). *Sand, water, silence: The embodiment of spirit, explorations in matter and psyche.* London: Jessica Kingsley Publishers.

Markman, K. D., Gavanski, S. J., & McMullen, M. N. (1993). The mental simulation of better and worse possible worlds. *Journal of Experimental Social Psychology, 29*, 87–109.

McKinney, K., & Kempson, D. A. (2012). Losing touch in social work practice. *Social Work, 57*(2), 189–191.

Mearns, D., & Thorne, B. (1998). *Person-centred counselling in action.* In W. Dryden (Ed., 2nd ed.). London: Sage Publications.

Milne, A. (2003). Teach yourself counselling. London: Hodder & Stoughton Ltd.

Montague, A. (1971). *Touching: The human significance of the skin.* New York: Harper & Row.

Montague, A. (1986). *Touching: The human significance of the skin.* London: HarperCollins.

Moy, C. (1981). Touch in the counselling relationship: an exploratory study. *Patient Counselling and Health Education, 3*(3), 89–94.

Phelan, J. E. (2009). Exploring the use of touch in the psychotherapeutic setting: A phenomenological review. *Psychotherapy, Research, Practice, Training, 46*(1), 97–111.

Proust, M. (1908). *Remembrance of things past.* www.age-of-the-sage.org/ Retrieved
11 April 2021.

Reeck, C., Ames, D. R., & Ochsner, K. N. (2016). The social regulation of emotion: An
integrative, cross-disciplinary model. *Trends in Cognitive Sciences, 20*(1), 47–63.

Smith, E. W. L., Clance, P. R., & Imes, S. (1998). *Touch in psychotherapy: Theory,
research, and practice.* New York: Guildford Press.

Strozier, A., Krizek, C., & Sale, K. (2010). Touch: Its use in psychotherapy. *Journal
of Social Work Practice: Psychotherapeutic Approaches in Health, Welfare and the
Community*, 17(1), 49–62.

Turner, B. A. (2005). *The handbook of sandplay therapy.* Cloverdale, California:
Temenos Press.

Routasala, P. (2001). Physical touch in nursing studies: A literature review. *JAN: Leading
Global Nursing Research, 30*(4), 843–850.

Thurschwell, P. (2009). *Sigmund Freud.* Retrieved from *file:///Users/doreenfleet/
Downloads/Pamela%20Thurschwell%20Sigmund%20Freud%202009%20(1).pdf*

Weiten, W., & Lloyd M. A. (2008). *Psychology applied to modern life* (9th ed.).
Wadsworth: Cengage Learning.

Williams, M. H. (1997). Boundary violations: Do some contended standards of care
fail to encompass commonplace procedures of humanistic, behavioral, and eclectic
psychotherapies? *Psychotherapy: Theory, Research, Practice, Training, 34*, 238–249.
https://doi.org/10.1037/h0087717

Wolberg, L. (1972) *The technique of psychotherapy.* New York: Grune and Stratton.

Wright, J. D. (2020). Training issues related to touch in counselling. *The Journal of
Counselor Preparation and Supervision, 13*(1). http://doi.org/10.7729/131.1340

Chapter 6

Structured sand-tray sessions

A goal without a plan is just a wish
(Antoine de Saint-Exupery [1900–1944] www.goodreads.com)

Intrapsychic experience, a significant feature in sand-tray therapy, fits with an unstructured approach with the client working creatively with symbols and metaphor. However, sometimes a client may ask for guidance to provide some initial plan to help them engage with the sand tray before working at depth intrapsychically.

As such, offering a structured sand-tray session can meet their request. Collaboration between client and therapist is essential in pluralistic therapy, so when a client asks for direction, it is necessary to respond so that their autonomy is respected. In addition, the therapist's active response is likely to increase the client's confidence, helping them continue contributing to any decision made throughout therapy.

Facilitating a structured sand-tray session can be likened to Vygotsky's (1978) 'zone of proximal development' that portrays the distinction between what a learner can do independently compared to what they can do with the help of an able individual. The support provided relates to 'scaffolding' (Vygotsky, 1978), describing how the supporting activity helps the learner complete a task. The term 'scaffolding' is a metaphor for the support removed in parts, as scaffolding in building construction is when the building can support itself. Copple and Bredekamp (2009) suggested that scaffolding could involve providing hints, adapting an activity or modelling a skill, with the 'scaffolding' removed once the learner has developed their skills and can complete the task independently (Vygotsky 1978).

In structured sand-tray therapy, the guidance on how to begin a session can be likened to scaffolding as once the client becomes more at ease using the sand tray, they can progress onto a more unstructured free-flowing process, taking the lead and setting the agenda for each session. The therapist's guidance can

DOI: 10.4324/9781003158707-6

help shift the responsibility from the client to a shared process when new to sand-tray therapy, communicating that 'we are doing this together'. However, even with such guidance, the sand tray still serves as a metaphorical experiential theatre. The client will need reassurance that there is no right way and no wrong way to work with the sand tray; whatever works for them is best.

As a therapist using sand tray, I find that some clients want to try this way of working but lack confidence at first; so offering guidance can help. However, a shift becomes evident when the same client walks into the therapy room and immediately begins to prepare the sand by flattening it or roughing it, or selecting objects without direction. This behaviour change indicates that the client is more at ease and ready to take the lead, directing the session from the start.

Ideas for structured sand-tray sessions

When clients struggle to start using the sand tray, they may ask or look to the therapist for guidance on how to begin. The therapist could ask a question such as, 'So what was the reason you came to therapy?' or 'What is it that makes you worry/sad/angry/hurt/distressed?' The therapist and the client will have discussed the client's goals and expectations before the first session, and by attending to them in the moment, the therapist will be able to identify the emotion most applicable for that client, used in the question above.

Life space

The client may state, 'there are so many problems, I'm so exhausted with it all, I just can't cope'. The therapist might then guide the client by asking them to select objects to represent the things in their life, making them distressed and feeling that they cannot cope. Once the client has finished selecting objects, the therapist can suggest dividing the sand around the objects representing each difficulty, indicating how much space each takes up in their life (using their finger or an object to draw the spaces around the objects). The therapist can then facilitate the client to talk about each, helping them to express their feelings. A helpful question asked once the client has explored their distress is, 'Where is the space for you in all this?' so that they can begin to offer self-compassion.

A second helpful follow-up question is 'What do you need to do to make space for some enjoyment/peace/quiet for yourself?' Even if the client responds with 'I have too much responsibility, and I can't change that', it can still help them recognise that they have needs too. The client may become more self-affirming and might consider communicating to other people in their life that they need some self-care in order to meet all their responsibilities.

Overall picture

A client might have a tendency to focus only on the negative things in their life, and the positive events in their life can become unnoticed, giving a distorted picture that their life is predominantly painful, difficult, and stressful. A therapist who becomes aware of this pattern in the client can help them get a sense of the overall picture of their life. Using the sand tray, the therapist can suggest that the client make a display by dividing the sand tray into two, using objects to represent the good things in their life for which they are thankful and the bad things causing them distress (or if the client prefers, creating two separate trays).

The client who is helped to talk about both good and bad can bring a sense of perspective for them.

Looking back at happier times

A client may state, 'I am never happy, I'm always scared, don't even know why really, just can't bring any enthusiasm for anything'. The therapist could ask the client if there was a time when they were happy, and if the client responds with the answer yes, the therapist might suggest, 'so when things were different in the past, what about making a display of the things that brought you joy, before this sadness/fear occurred?'

After the client has finished creating the sand display and explored it, it might be appropriate to ask, 'Is there anything in the sand tray that is missing in your life today?' Sometimes, the client can make a change to bring something back, which gave them joy in the past. I have experience of clients who say things such as 'I used to read a lot', 'I used to go to church', or 'I used to exercise regularly' and decided to bring that back into their lives once again to see if they can regain some of that happiness. Some adults can be so weighed down with responsibility and caring for others that they forget what brought them joy in the past, and this exercise can be a reminder that they need some self-care too.

Eight emotions

A client may avoid talking about their emotions and, when feelings begin to emerge, revert to their thinking as they talk. It can help if the therapist gives the client some guidance to connect to their emotions and feelings.

Paul Ekman (1972) claimed that there are six basic "emotions of happiness, surprise, fear, sadness, anger and disgust, combined with contempt" (Ekman, 1992, p. 550). Later research by various scholars (Ekman & Friesen, 1986, 1988; Ekman & Heider, 1988; Izard & Haynes, 1988: Ricci Bitti et al., 1988) suggested one addition by distinguishing contempt from disgust. Other researchers (Tomkins & McCarter, 1964; Izard, 1971) argued that interest and shame exist as emotions within culture. However, whatever the emotion, helping a client explore and express their feelings linked to their distress is a significant feature of humanistic therapy.

Patel and Patel (2019) discussed how the inhibition of emotional expression could "endanger our health, both physically and psychologically, including our well being" (p. 16). Furthermore, they argued that individuals who have difficulty managing their emotions risk developing certain behaviours, including substance abuse, eating disorders, and abnormal sleep patterns (Patel & Patel, 2019). Similarly, Cote (2005) argued that continued repression of emotion in the workplace leads to stress, causing increased heart rate and anxiety. Finally, Pennebaker (1997) agreed how continued repression of emotions could suppress a person's immunity, making them vulnerable to conditions ranging from the common cold virus to cancer.

Therefore, "expressing one's true emotions and the associated feelings are crucial to physical health, mental health and general well being" (Patel & Patel, 2019, p. 20); in contrast, consistent repression of emotions can lead to physical and psychological ill-health. Talking with a therapist can help a person explore and express what they have been trying to avoid, which can be beneficial.

Greenberg (2001) argued that emotion has a significant role in bringing therapeutic change. Therefore, a therapist needs to allow and accept a client's emotional pain so they can move towards healing (Greenberg et al., 1998).

Working creatively, such as using the sand tray in therapy, can bring relief or facilitate catharsis (Runco, 2014). Furthermore, Hirt (1999) suggested, "individuals in positive mood states have been shown to be more creative ..." (p. 241), adding to the argument that creativity in therapy is a resource that can bring benefits for clients.

In the Eight emotions sand-tray session, the therapist invites the client to select objects related to any of the eight emotions and place them in the sand tray:

- Anger
- Disgust
- Fear
- Happiness
- Sadness
- Contempt
- Surprise
- Shame
  - Alternatively, another emotion that is significant for the client (such as envy, jealousy, love, tenderness, or emotion they name using their own words can be used. For example, 'Mr Grumpy', 'Bitchy Bessy', 'Happy Harry').

The therapist will need to stay alongside the client and hold an attitude without judgment or expectation, facilitating them to explore and express this emotion and the feelings associated with the related experience.

Alternatively, the therapist could invite the client to divide the sand tray into two or more emotions, exploring and expressing them in turn.

Relationship dynamics and associated emotions

Until the 1980s, most research on human emotion focused on the individual by taking a cognitive stance (Manstead, https://thepsychologist.bps.org.uk/volume-18/edition-8/social-dimension-emotion retrieved January 2020). However, Scherer et al. (1986) suggested that emotion is more likely to be linked socially with others than an individual phenomenon. Although some emotions linked to non-social objects exist, such as fear of heights, emotions like affection, sympathy, compassion, and admiration depend on others being present physically or psychologically (Manstead, 2020). Another point made by Manstead concerns the point that people seek others to share emotion, supporting the social link.

A client may refer to difficulties in their significant relationships, blaming themselves for the problematic dynamics or continue to blame others. It can help if the therapist suggests exploring the client's emotions borne from those challenging relationships. Relationship dynamics vary incredibly, and a wide range of emotions may be experienced, including shame, hurt, anger, humiliation, disempowerment, frustration, love, tenderness, dependence, responsibility, pride, togetherness, exclusion, desperation, fear, and/or feeling abused or ostracised. The therapist will need to stay alongside the client to work with whatever the client brings to the session.

My givers and takers

A therapist could suggest that the client might want to work on significant relationships, by first selecting an object to represent them and placing it in the middle of the sand tray. Sunderland (1993) created an activity called 'The Givers and the Takers', used "to heighten the awareness of the concept of support" (p. 120), which members of the public can use to become more emotionally literate. Therefore, taking a similar approach, a client in therapy is asked, 'who in your life do you see as givers and takers", helping them explore a problematic relationship – an expanded explanation of this question is 'givers being the people who help you feel happy and takers being people who leave you feeling down or negative in some way'.

The client could then be guided further by the therapist suggesting, "you could try selecting objects for those you see as 'givers and takers' in your life and place them in the sand in relation to the object representing you". For example, a person may feel drained and diminished by certain relationships and rejuvenated by others, and some may experience both in the same relationship at different times. It could be that a client may have the perception that a balance between giving and taking is acceptable, and the problem might be that they perceive the other always to be the taker or always the giver. This focus can help explore the dynamics from the client's perspective, indicating a possible need for change in a relationship.

However, it may also be appropriate to suggest that the client may want to shift the focus, exploring if they are a giver or a taker in certain relationships. Here they are helped to focus on how they might impact the relationship and use the symbolic objects to represent this. Again, to always be the giver or always be the taker can be problematic. For example, a persistent giver does not allow the other to give, which has its own rewards even if that is just a good feeling of offering something to the relationship. In contrast, to be the consistent taker can be a selfish attitude, taking the other for granted on a regular basis. This perspective can indicate that it may be the client who needs to make changes so that the relationship becomes a more reciprocal one.

The therapist will need to respond to the usual cues such as the client's words, tone and pace of voice, and body language; the symbolic objects and what they represent; and the spatial arrangement.

The spatial arrangement in this exercise can be significant, indicating how influential the other person is on the client's emotions and frame of mind, which can be positive or distressing, or a combination of the two. Thus, in addition to helping the client express their thoughts on the dynamics of the targeted relationship, the therapist will also need to help them explore and express their feelings. Greenberg (2004) argued that emotional intelligence has an "optimal adaptation, which involves an integration of reason and emotion" (p. 3).

Speaking the unspoken: unfinished business

Sometimes, a client may want to focus on something they needed to say to another person but did not, resulting in distress due to a sense of unfinished business. The reason for this can vary, such as them feeling disempowered, them not wanting to hurt the other person's feelings, or that the other person is no longer present. For example, a client may experience unresolved emotion after a bereavement and respond to the question of 'what is the hardest thing about your loss by saying?':

'I never got the chance to tell them this …'
'I've lost my chance to tell them …'
'At the time, I just couldn't say it to them …'
'I wish I could tell them …'

Korb et al. (1989) described how unresolved experiences are incomplete and "draw energy away from present functioning, thus inhibiting the ability of the individual to participate fully in present experiences" (p. 85). Greenberg and Malcolm (2002) stated, "helping clients to work through unresolved emotional experiences with significant others has a long and important history in psychotherapy" (p. 406). The unresolved emotion may lead to anxiety, anger, resentment, hurt, or guilt. Sunderland (1993) created a paper exercise on unfinished business to help people "become aware of the unresolved feelings (the unfinished business)" (p. 112) they have with others, which can be used as an individual exercise or in a group.

Perls et al. (1951) argued that avoidance of painful feelings in therapy was a key factor in the persistence of unfinished business. Such persistence of a painful unresolved issue can result in the client becoming "psychologically and/or emotionally stuck" (Greenberg & Malcolm, 2002, p. 406). However, in sand-tray therapy, the client's experience is "transferred from the inner world to the outer world and made visible" (Kalff, 2003), and the symbolic objects help the client connect and express their emotions.

Greenberg and Safran (1987) suggested that empty-chair work could bring change for the client regarding this issue. In this intervention, the client guided to visualise the deceased sitting in the empty chair can then engage in an imaginary dialogue with them. Greenberg (2001) suggested that the therapist would then facilitate the client to reflect on their emotional reactions, leading to relief and resolution due to them speaking the unspoken. Greenberg et al. (1993) argued that resolution of unfinished business using the empty-chair dialogue results in the client moving away "from expressing blame, complaint, and/or hurt" (Greenberg & Malcolm, 2002, p. 407) to a state where they can acknowledge and establish an interpersonal need. Furthermore, the client may become more self-affirming, forgive the other, or hold others accountable (Greenberg et al., 1993).

Brown (1990) suggested an intervention akin to Greenberg et al. (1993) approach by facilitating a guided imaginary conversation with the deceased by asking questions such as, "what is it you want to say to them"? The empty chair is not used here, but the client can still express what they needed to say to the deceased in the presence of an empathic listener.

A similar approach can use the sand tray, with the object representing the deceased placed in the sand, and the client helped to act out and speak the unspoken, projecting onto the object representing the person they need to converse with. The client is free to use additional objects to represent specific experiences related to their unfinished business. The client will most likely experience a sense of relief having spoken out loud what had been unspoken and combined with the therapist as an empathic listener, and experience a phenomenological shift regarding this issue.

References

Brown, J. C. (1990). Loss and grief: An overview and guided imagery intervention model. *Journal of Mental Health Counseling, 12*(4), 434–445.

Copple, C., & Bredekamp, S. (2009). *Developmentally appropriate practice in childhood programs*. Washington, DC: National Association for the Education of Young Children.

Cote, S. (2005). A social interaction model of the effects of emotion regulation on work strain. *Academy of Management Review, 30*, 509–530.

Ekman, P. (1992). Are there basic emotions? *Psychology Review, 99*(3), 550–553.

Ekman, P., & Friesen, W. V. (1986). A new pan-cultural expression of emotion. *Motivation and Emotion, 10*, 159–168.

Ekman, P., & Friesen, W. V. (1988). Who knows what about contempt: A reply to Izard and Haynes. *Motivation and Emotion, 12*, 17–22.

Ekman, P., & Friesen, W. V., & Ellsworth, P. (1972). *Emotion in the human face: Guidelines for research and an integration of findings*. New York: Pergamon Press.

Ekman, P., & Heider, K. G. (1988). The universality of a contempt expression: A replication. *Motivation and Emotion, 12*, 303–308.

Greenberg, L. S. (2001). *Emotion-focused therapy. Coaching clients to work through their feelings*. Washington, DC: American Psychological Association.

Greenberg, L. S. (2004). Emotion-focused therapy. *Clinical Psychology & Psychotherapy, 11*, 3–16.

Greenberg, L. S., & Malcolm, W. (2002). Resolving unfinished business: Relating process to outcome. *Journal of Consulting and Clinical Psychology, 70*(2), 406–416.

Greenberg, L. S., & Rice, L., & Elliott, R. (1993). *Facilitating emotional change: The moment by moment process*. New York: Guilford Press.

Greenberg, L. S., & Safran, J. (1987). *Emotion in psychotherapy: Affect, cognition and the process of change*. New York: Guilford Press.

Greenberg, L. S., Watson, J., & Lietaer, G. (1998). *Handbook of experiential therapy*. New York: Guilford Press.

Hirt, E. R. (1999). Mood. In M. A. Runco & S. R. Pritzker (Eds.). *Encyclopedia of creativity*. Vol. *2*, pp. 241–250. San Diego, CA: Academic Press.

Izard, C. (1971). *The face of emotion*. New York: Appleton-Century-Crofts.

Izard, C., & Haynes, O. M. (1988). On the form and universality of the contempt expression: A challenge to Ekman and Friesen's claim of discovery. *Motivation and Emotion, 12*, 1–16.

Kalff, D. (2003). *Sandplay: A psychotherapeutic approach to the psyche*. Cloverdale, CA: Temenos Press.

Korb, M., & Gorrell, J., & Van de Riet, V. (1989). *Gestalt Therapy*. Oxford: Pergamon Press.

Manstead, A. S. R. (2020). The social dimension of emotion. *The British Psychological Society*. https://thepsychologist.bps.org.uk/volume-18/edition-8/social-dimension-emotion Retrieved 12/1/2020

Patel, J., & Patel, P. (2019). Consequences of repression of emotion: Physical health, mental health and general well being. *International Journal of Psychotherapy Practice and Research, 1*(3), 16–21.

Pennebaker, J. W. (1997). *Opening up: The healing power of expressing emotion*. New York: Guildford Press.

Perls, F., & Hefferline, R., & Goodman, P. (1951). *Gestalt therapy*. New York: Delta.

Ricci Bitti, P. E., Brighetti, G., Garotti, P., & Boggi-Cavallo, P. (1988, August). *Is contempt expressed by pan-cultural facial movements?* Paper presented at the XXIV International Congress of Psychology, Sydney, Australia.

Runco, M. A. (2014). *Creativity: Theories and Themes: Research, development, and practice*. London, UK and Waltham, USA: Elsevier Inc.

Scherer, K. R., & Wallbott, H., & Summerfield, A. B. (1986). *Experiencing emotion*. Cambridge: Cambridge University Press.

Sunderland, M. (1993). *Draw on your emotions*. Bicester, Oxon: Winslow Press Ltd.

Tomkins, S. S., & McCarter, R. (1964). What and where are the primary affects? Some evidence for a theory. *Perceptual and Motor Skills, 18*, 119–158.

Vygotsky, L. S. (1978). *Mind in society: The development of higher psychosocial processes*. Cambridge, MA: Harvard University Press.

Chapter 7

Particular challenges for sand-tray therapy

Facing it, always facing it, that's the way to get through
(Conrad, 1986. www.amazon.co.uk/)

Therapists who intend to offer sand-tray therapy are faced with a number of challenges. Such challenges will need to be faced head-on and managed to overcome possible blocks and help clients engage with therapy. In addition, specific practical requirements will need addressing, with resources acquired taking some time to collect.

Cutting through intellectualisation as a defence

Stewart (2013) defined *intellectualisation* as the "deliberate avoidance of dealing with feelings by filtering and analysing everything through head logic" (p. 471).

Stewart (2013) discussed how intellectualisation is a defence mechanism, a "flight manoeuvre" to avoid feeling stressed or anxious. Sometimes, clients in therapy can engage in intellectualisation and rationalisation as a defence against expressing their feelings. In sand-tray therapy, feelings can emerge very quickly when exploring symbolic meanings, and when touching both objects and sand, intellectualisation can disrupt any therapeutic progress, challenging the therapist.

Howard (2006) described how "the defence of intellectualisation is a way of keeping both" the therapist and the client's "own feelings at a distance." (p. 18). However, defences can be helpful to an individual as a way of functioning in the world (Stewart, 2013). For example, it may be useful to avoid expressing anger in the workplace to avoid overt conflict, but defences can sometimes become problematic for individuals who continue to avoid their emotions. When avoidance becomes a habit in therapy, the client who continues to resist expressing a feeling linked to a particular issue (Howard, 2006) is likely to experience a block in the therapeutic process. The therapist

DOI: 10.4324/9781003158707-7

will need to help the client work with this resistance and use challenges to help the client get in touch with their feelings and emotions in the session.

Runco (2014) suggested how working creatively could bring a shift in perspective, "making it easy to break routine and find original ideas and solutions" (p. 340). Such exploration can contribute to greater personal understanding, and "one of the best things a person can do is to maintain health is to find opportunities for self-expression" (Runco, 2014, p. 121).

In 1961, Rogers argued that counsellors "have a responsibility to offer safe, accepting relationships that will foster constructive creativity within clients" (Lawrence et al., 2015, p. 168). Delivering sand-tray therapy is conducive to Rogers's expectation as it establishes a creative environment for the client to express their thoughts and feelings using the media of sand and symbolic objects. Gladding (2008) went further regarding the importance of creativity in therapy and stated how past strategies are not always appropriate and "if counseling is to continue to be on the forefront of the helping professions, it must continue to promote creativity" (p. 103).

Working creatively by using the sand tray involves the symbolic representation of experience, helping the client connect to their feelings. As the client engages in the visual and tactile process of seeing and touching the objects and sand, this shifts the client into a direct experience involving physical sensation, emotion, and thinking.

Badenoch (2008) suggested how using the sand tray makes it more difficult for the client to stay with their thinking alone. Homeyer and Sweeney (2011) supported this argument and stated how "sand-tray therapy may cut through the defences" (p. 11) of intellectualisation and rationalisation.

Sand-tray therapy is likely to bring benefits even for clients who tend to be more rational in their expression. The sand-tray process and the therapist's empathic presence are therapeutically powerful in that it challenges the client to connect with their feelings and thoughts. Averill (1999) stated, "On the border between cognition and emotion lies creativity" (p. 765). Gutbezahl and Averill (1996) argued, "… emotions themselves may be the product of a creative process" (In Runco 2014, p. 114), contributing to the significance of creativity in therapy.

However, it is likely to be challenging for a client who has a habit of avoiding their feelings when engaged in therapy, which "calls emotions into the room" (Hass-Cohen, 2008, p. 293). Harrington et al. (1983) argued that unconditional positive regard (Rogers, 1957; Mearns & Thorne, 1999; Merry, 2002) was essential when offering creative interventions in therapy so that the client feels respected and appreciated, making it more likely that they will take a risk and try something new.

In her initial assessment, Jackie (Fleet, 2019) was well aware of her tendency to intellectualise and identified one of her goals as wanting to stay with her emotions and express her feelings. She asked for my support to challenge her whenever she moved away from her feelings and began to rationalise.

Jackie believed this would be useful, so we agreed that I would try to refocus her away from her thoughts and back to her feelings. However, the symbolic objects also contribute to helping a client stay with their feelings.

The shark object Jackie placed in the sand acted as a phenomenological hook and aided unconscious material to emerge relating to her fear. I asked Jackie a Socratic question concerning the shark's symbolism that enabled her to stay with her fear (Chapter 3). She was able to express this powerful emotion, bringing insight, owning her fear.

Persistence of the adult persona as a block

May (1975/1994) defined *creativity* as "the process of bringing something new into being"(p. 37), so this understanding could indicate the benefits of working creatively in therapy that could bring new perception and insight for the client. However, some adults may be reluctant to using creative methods, including sand tray in therapy. Malchiodi (2005) suggested that adults might shy away from working creatively because they perceive themselves as not imaginative or anxious about self-expression. Besides, the adult persona does not fit easily with working creatively, as a client with this attitude may view this as childlike play.

Adams (1974) suggested that playfulness in adulthood is frowned upon in the United States, creating a cultural block to original thinking. The general view by adult society being "if an adult has a problem, they should be serious about solving it" (Runco, 2014, p. 279). This view could be specifically relevant to adult clients who have introjected society's expectations to behave as responsible adults. They are likely to view themselves as needing to think seriously about solving their difficulties and, as adults, should control their emotions regarding a specific issue. Thus, they "may be inhibited in their spontaneity in therapy" (Malchiodi, 2005, p. 13) and resist creativity due to the learned rules about self-expression of the adult persona.

Gardner (1993) suggested how creative people demonstrate spontaneity, inhibition, and authenticity and are viewed as playful and often childlike. Furthermore, Kaplan (2014) interviewed Harriet Friedman, who argued how modern society does not value the irrational, play, spontaneity, or unconscious, which could discourage creative interventions in therapy, especially for adults.

A further block to working creatively in therapy could be due to the myth of left and right brain differences between people (Allen & van der Zwan, 2019). Sperry (1961, 1968) argued how the hemispheres in the human brain have different functions.

Over time, the notion that people use their left brain for thinking and logic and their right brain for creativity and intuition led to the fallacy that people are more left-brained or right-brained thinkers. However, Burgess (2020) stated, "The theory that a person is either left-brained or right-brained is not supported by scientific research" (www.medicalnewstoday.com/articles/321037. Retrieved 23 March 2021).

Nielsen et al. (2013) also argued that there is no evidence to suggest that this is the case and that the left-brain-right-brain argument is outdated. Current neuroscience research suggests creativity involves cross-brain pattern activity between the left and right brain hemispheres (Park et al., 2016). However, the myth that the right side of the brain is creative and the left associated with the intellect persists. Allen and van der Zwan (2019) stated, "the idea of right- or left-brain learning is possibly one of the oldest and most pervasive neuromyths circulating today" (p. 192). Therefore, if an adult client presents for therapy with the perception that they are more left-brained and intellectual, they may be averse to engaging in any creative method to explore their issue. Furthermore, the therapist is likely to be challenged when aiming to help the client connect with their feelings, exploring the metaphors and symbolism in their discourse.

Homeyer and Sweeney (2011) suggested that the best way to respond to an adult client who views sand-tray work as too juvenile, vague, and "unserious" is to acknowledge their uncomfortable feelings and suggest they experiment and have a go. Such an approach would be supplemented with the reassurance that there is no expectation to stay with it and communicate that they can stop at any time. Homeyer and Sweeney argue that this is like giving the client permission to try something new, which they would not normally do, and many clients will try it out.

Turner (2005) also discussed how sometimes adults enter the therapy room and, seeing the objects, state, "Oh ... I see you work with children" (p. 363). Turner's (2005) usual response would be to suggest that sand-tray could be used with adults to help them explore deeper issues. Turner also suggested informing the client that "It is simply a way of allowing what is inside us, the stuff that doesn't have words, to come up and out in symbols" (p. 364). Furthermore, Turner (2005) often engaged in an explicit demonstration of using the sand tray and objects, suggesting that the client can use wet or dry sand. However, she described how she would strongly challenge a reluctant client by voicing her opinion that she believed it would be beneficial and that they may want to seriously consider using it.

A person-centred therapy (PCT) therapist using sand tray would question making such a solid challenge to the client as they believe that the client is the expert of their own pain, knows what direction to take, and sets the agenda (Rogers, 1961). Therefore, the PCT therapist would not try to persuade the client to work in a particular way.

However, a repost to this criticism may be that an experienced therapist of creative methods might argue that sometimes adults cannot overcome a block alone and need direction to help them master their reluctance.

Then once able to engage, the creative process can provide a unique perspective on their issue. Runco (2014) discussed how both Rogers (1961; 1995) and Maslow (1971) linked creativity to self-actualisation, tying it to psychological health. The tendency for the playfulness of creative people "may be a reflection of their spontaneity and self-actualization" (Runco, 2014, p. 279), so it may be that helping clients to engage in creative work in therapy may bring other benefits.

I have worked with both men and women who are often surprised when I suggest they might want to try working with the sand tray. I find the following comment goes a long way in meeting the expectations of the adult persona:

> So you know how we often using metaphor in our language to describe our experience? We might say, 'I feel so confused, I'm all at sea' or 'I have so much responsibility, I feel like a little donkey carrying a heavy load up a hill'. Here the objects act as physical metaphors to represent your thoughts and feelings, and their symbolism can really help you to begin exploring your issue in a deeper way. Working this way is about helping you explore your thoughts and your emotions.

The reminder that they will most likely use metaphor in their speech and to give concrete examples seems to satisfy the adult client how working this way is appropriate for them. There have been numerous times when I have counselled adult clients who have expressed surprise at the power of working with the sand tray and the insight gained. Expressing their feelings linked to a previously guarded experience often results in a phenomenological shift regarding their perceptions and feelings.

Male gender role socialisation as a block

Good and Robertson (2010) suggested that most men are socialised to work on their problems cognitively, which could contribute to male clients being more resistant to work creatively in therapy than female clients. Pederson and Vogel (2007) took a similar stance, arguing that men are more willing to engage in therapy when focusing on cognitions rather than emotions. Hass-Cohen (2008) suggests how sand-tray therapy is associated with emotional expression, so there may be more reluctance from some male clients who are uncomfortable when expressing their feelings. Pattee and Farber (2008) suggested that men could feel more exposed and vulnerable when revealing strong feelings than women do.

However, even when supported with research, such arguments may still be criticised by some by stating how such assertions are gender stereotypical. The PCT stance would be to avoid making any prior assumptions no matter what a client's gender and aim to stay within their own unique frame of reference. However, it may be helpful for a therapist to be aware of the possible impact of role socialisation regarding male clients who tend to avoid their feelings. The male client may be more open to change if they feel respected, and then the therapist may offer congruency and challenge to help free them from such powerful expectations.

It might also be helpful to establish rapport with male clients so that they feel more at ease. Also, it can help to accept and stay alongside them when they need to engage in some discourse on setting the context of a particular issue and discuss the facts around an experience until they are ready to engage in a more profound way.

This pre-phenomenological process (Fleet, 2019) can be a necessary precursor before they become engaged in the phenomenological process of exploring their intrapsychic experience.

Adequate resources required for sand-tray therapy

There are practical requirements, which need to be addressed prior to offering pluralistic sand-tray therapy. Besides the usual resources such as counselling contracts, personal information sheets, clinical assessment forms, and therapy information sheets for new clients, specific resources will need to be gathered.

Firstly, a large enough tray for the client to work fluidly and with enough space to create a sand display without feeling too restricted will need to be sourced.

The sand tray I use with clients is wooden and measures 65cm × 45cm. However, some therapists use smaller trays successfully, so it is a matter of personal choice. Good advice is to have a sand tray with a lid so that you can keep the tray clean, and it is wise to use play-sand that is both fine and clean. Also, there needs to be a large enough table to hold the sand tray and selected objects before being placed in the sand. A comfortable chair that fits neatly with the table of appropriate height will be necessary and the usual counselling chairs.

There also needs to be a range of good quality symbolic objects arranged in a cabinet or on shelves in the therapy room. It is useful to provide a small basket or a box so that the client can use this to place the objects during the selection process. Small toys are acceptable for children, but for adults, I would advise collecting quality objects. I have collected objects from visiting different places at home and abroad, including specialised sand-tray online retailers, local shops, charity stores, jumble sales, model shops, and beaches (stones and shells), and have been given objects by other people to add to my collection. However, it is essential to realise that you cannot provide an object for every single issue. My experience is that if the client cannot find a particular object to represent a particular issue, they will use an abstract object and make it fit.

An example is taken from the case study with Jackie (Fleet, 2019) when she wanted to use an object to represent her sports car, and the car object on the shelf did not fit with her symbolism. So instead, she selected an object of a shark and satisfyingly placed it in the sand describing how fast it was. It will probably take some time to build a good range of objects, and the list below can give you some idea of the type of objects to begin collecting.

- Diverse human objects – representing different:
  - Races
  - Ages
  - Disabilities
  - Fictional characters
  - Person expressing different emotions:
    - For example, anger, sadness, joy, love
- Animals
  - Power animals (e.g., tiger, lion, bear)
  - Gentle animals (e.g., lamb, mouse)
  - Domesticated animals (e.g., dog, cat)
- Insects
  - Spider
  - Scorpion
- Reptiles
  - Snake
  - Crocodile
  - Alligator
- Fantasy creatures
  - Monsters
  - Dragons
- Religious/spiritual objects
  - Angels
  - Cherubs
- Nature
  - Trees
  - Flowers
  - Mountain
  - Stones
  - Crystals
- Man-made objects
  - Wishing well
  - Birds cage
  - Lighthouse
  - House
  - Ship
  - Car
  - Bike
- Abstract objects
  - Hearts
  - Ball of string

- Stones
- Shells
- Beads
- Small bricks

In addition to building up a good range of objects, I have found a lamp to be a helpful resource that lights up the sand tray, giving an excellent focus for the client to work. Some clients will want to sculpt the sand into valleys and hills, and wet sand is easier to work with. Having water available in a jug or a spray bottle gives the client a choice to work with dry or wet sand. A tool that can be used to smooth, rake, or dig holes in the sand can also be a good addition, and some therapists will paint the bottom of the sand-tray blue so that a client can create an image of an island surrounded by sea if they should want to. Finally, clients will want to clean their hands during or after the session, so cleansing wipes are a good resource to have available, as is an iPhone to take photographs of the sand displays.

References

Adams, J. (1974). *Conceptual blockbusting.* New York: W. W. Norton.

Allen, K., & van der Zwan, R. (2019). The myth of left- vs right-brain learning. *International Journal of Innovation, Creativity and Change,* 5(1) 189–200.

Averill, R. J. (1999). Creativity in the domain of emotion. In T. Dalgleish & M. J. Power (Eds.), *Handbook of cognition and emotion* (pp. 765–782). New York: John Wiley & Sons.

Badenoch, B. (2008). *Being a brain-wise therapist: A practical guide to interpersonal neurobiology.* London: W. W. Norton.

Burgess, L. (2020). Left brain vs. right brain: Fact and fiction. Medical News Today. (www.medicalnewstoday.com/articles/321037. Retrieved 23 March 2021).

Conrad, J. (1986). *Typhoon.* New York: Oxford University Press. (Kindle DX version). www.amazon.co.uk

Fleet, D. (2019). *Transformation hidden in the sand: Developing a theoretical framework using a sand-tray intervention with adult clients.* Doctoral thesis. Staffordshire University. Stoke-on-Trent. Available from Ethos STORE – Staffordshire Online Repository. https://eprints.staffs.ac.uk/id/eprint/5763

Gardner, H. (1993). *Creating minds: An anatomy of creativity seen through the lives of Freud, Einstein, Picasso, Stravinsky, Eliot, Graham, and Gandhi.* New York: Basic Books.

Gladding, S. T. (2008). The impact of creativity in counselling. *Journal of Creativity in Mental Health,* 3, 97–104.

Good, G. E., & Robertson, J. M. (2010). To accept a pilot? Addressing men's ambivalence and altering their expectancies about therapy. *Psychotherapy Theory, Research, Practice Training,* 47(3), 306–315. doi 10.1037/a0021162.

Gutbezahl, J., & Averill, R. J. (1996). Individual differences in emotional creativity as manifested in words and pictures. *Creativity Research Journal,* 9, 327–337.

Harrington, D. M., Block, J., & Block, J. H. (1983). Predicting creativity in preadolescence form divergent thinking in early childhood. *Journal of Personality and Social Psychology, 45*, 609–623.

Hass-Cohen, N. (2008). CREATE: Art Therapy Relational Neuroscience Principles (ATR-N). In N. Hass-Cohen & R. Carr (Eds.), *Art therapy and clinical neuroscience.* London: Jessica Kingsley Publishers.

Homeyer, L. E., & Sweeney, D. S. (2011). *Sandtray therapy: A practical manual* (2nd ed.). London: Routledge.

Howard, S. (2006). Psychodynamic counselling in a nutshell. In W. Dryden (Ed.), *Counselling in a nutshell series.* London: Sage Publications.

Kaplan, J. (2014). A conversation with Harriet Friedman. *Journal of Sandplay Therapy, 23*(1), 7–20.

Lawrence, C., & Foster, V. A., & Tieso, C. L. (2015). Creating creative clinicians: Incorporating creativity into counselor education. *Journal of Creativity in Mental Health, 10*, 166–180.

Malchiodi, C. (2005). *Expressive therapies.* New York: Guildford Press.

Maslow, A. H. (1971). *The farther reaches of human nature.* New York: Viking.

May, R. (1975/1994). *The courage to create.* New York: W. W. Norton.

Mearns, D., & Thorne, B. (1999). *Person-centred counselling in action* (2nd ed.). In W. Dryden (Ed.). London: Sage.

Merry, T. (2002). *Learning and being in person-centred counselling.* Ross-on-Wye: PCCS Books.

Nielsen, J. A., Zielinski, B. A., Ferguson, M. A., Lainhart, J. E., & Anderson, J. S. (2013). An evaluation of the left-brain vs. right-brain hypothesis with resting state functional connectivity magnetic resonance imaging. *PloS ONE, 8*(8), e71275.

Park, S., & Kim, K. K., & Hahm, J. (2016). Neuro-scientific studies of creativity. *Dementia and Neurocognitive Disorders, 15*(4), 110–114.

Pattee, D., & Farber, B. A. (2008). Patients' experience of self-disclosure in psychotherapy: The effects of gender and gender role identification. Psychotherapy Research, *18*(3), 306–315.

Pederson, E. L. & Vogel, D. L. (2007). Male gender role conflict and willingness to seek counseling: Testing a mediation model on college-aged men. *Journal of Counseling Psychology, 54*(4), 373–384. doi: 10.1037/0022-0167.54.4.373.

Rogers, C. R. (1957). The necessary and sufficient conditions of therapeutic personality change. *Journal of Consulting Psychology, 21*, 95–103.

Rogers, C. R. (1961). *On becoming a person.* Boston, MA: Houghton Mifflin.

Rogers, C. R. (1995). On becoming a person: A therapist's view of psychotherapy. Boston, MA: Houghton-Mifflin (Original work published in 1961).

Runco, M. A. (2014). *Creativity: Theories and themes: Research, development and practice* (2nd ed.). London: Elsevier.

Sperry, R. W. (1961). Cerebral organization and behavior. *Science, 133*, 1749–1757.

Sperry, R. W. (1968). Hemisphere deconnection and unity in conscious awareness. *American Psychologist, 28*, 723–733.

Stewart, W. (2013). *An A-Z of counselling theory and practice* (5th ed.). Hampshire: Cengage Learning EMEA.

Turner, B. A. (2005). *The handbook of sandplay therapy.* Cloverdale, CA: Temenos Press.

Chapter 8

Protocol for pluralistic sand-tray therapy

Let our advance worrying become advance thinking and planning.
(Sir Winston Churchill. www.goodreads.com)

This chapter will provide step-by-step guidance on how to deliver pluralistic sand-tray therapy. Instruction will provide detailed information on planning and managing the initial appointment, the first therapy session, continuing sessions, and the end session.

Initial assessment session

During the initial assessment of pluralistic sand-tray therapy, when a client arrives seeking help with their difficulties, it is vital to establish an empathic and collaborative relationship to facilitate an atmosphere of shared dialogue. After the initial introductions, the therapist will need to explain how sand-tray therapy works; done verbally and combined with an information sheet, it gives the prospective client clear information, making it easier for them to decide whether to go ahead with the therapy. They can take the information sheet away to refer to after the initial session and ask further questions before the first session begins. The expression below might be a helpful introduction, explaining how sand-tray therapy works:

> The aim of this therapy is for us to work together to help you meet your hopes and expectations from therapy and for us to decide what might work best for you. Sometimes it can be hard to find the right words to talk about what you need to, and the objects, acting as symbols, can help you do that. Sand-tray therapy can also help you work on those deeper, painful issues in a way where you can express your thoughts and feelings, and I will help and support you throughout the process.

It might help further if the therapist gives a short demonstration for the client by selecting an object and describing the symbolism from their perspective.

DOI: 10.4324/9781003158707-8

For example, they may choose an object of a donkey carrying a heavy load, place it in the sand, and say:

> So, for example, this object might symbolise someone who feels overwhelmed with responsibility, just like this little donkey carrying a heavy load. By exploring what the object represents, this way of working can help you open up and verbalise what you need to say.
>
> Many clients find they can express their thoughts and feelings and seem to find the "right" words to express what they had difficulty saying before therapy.

When working with the information sheet in the initial session, it is best to take a personable approach and provide the most relevant material so the client can make an informed choice in deciding to have therapy. A space to record the issue/s the client needs to focus on and a space to identify their "personal strengths and resources" (Cooper & McLeod, 2011 p. 184) will be needed. This information, gathered by a purposeful discussion, will contribute to establishing the tasks and methods for therapy.

The client is encouraged to contribute by being asked questions like, "How does this sound to you" and "What do you feel about working this way"? Any opportunity for purposeful discussion is taken, establishing a collaborative process. It is also crucial that the therapist is transparent when the potential client considers whether they want to go ahead with the therapy. This process needs to involve the therapist informing the client about other forms of help available so they can make an informed decision.

Cooper and Dryden (2016) discuss how O'Neill's (1999) research argued how a client involved in discussing available alternative helping professions contributed to strengthening the client's trust in the therapist.

Once an individual decides to go ahead with the therapy, then various procedures need to take place. A client information sheet will need to be completed, incorporating the client's personal contact details and health conditions that the therapist needs to know and how regular and long the therapy will be. Once again, this can be done collaboratively, especially concerning the length of therapy and session frequency, with both therapist and client coming to a shared agreement.

The client will be required to sign a consent form once informed about the therapist's ethical framework and confidentiality boundaries. In addition to the usual criteria on the consent form, there will need to be a section related explicitly to sand-tray therapy. For example, it is helpful to take photographs of sand displays for counselling supervision, and the client will need to agree to this. Clients can also benefit from taking photographs as they might find it helpful to refer to these during a session or take a copy home.

Clinical assessment and feedback viewed as essential features in pluralistic therapy (Cooper & McLeod, 2011) inform both the therapist and the client of what is working well and what might need to be changed. In terms of out-come measures, the therapist may have a favourite questionnaire they already use, such as CORE (Twigg & McInnes, 2010) or another preferred option.

It is also helpful to have a pre- and post-clinical assessment to compare any change in the client's level of distress by the end of therapy. Again, the client will need to give consent before therapy to complete this assessment. This feedback gives the client the power to express how effective they think it has been, providing essential information to the therapist concerning any required changes. To offer the client a chance to give their views, whether this is verbal, written, or a combination of both can be delivered collaboratively with shared dialogue.

When identifying the client's goals or expectations for therapy, it can be helpful "to invite the client to formulate specific goal statements as a means of anchoring therapy" (Cooper & Dryden, 2016, p. 19). Writing these down to be referred to during therapy can help keep the client remain focused on what they wanted to achieve. A Goals Form offered by Cooper and McLeod (2011, p. 189) can be used in the initial assessment with the client to write down their goals, or the therapist can hold the pen, writing down the client's answers to the questions.

However, the form may be amended partway through therapy to incorp-orate other goals that emerge.

For some clients, goals will remain unchanged, but for others, goals established in the initial assessment may change as the therapy progresses, or the client may identify new goals. For example, a client may begin therapy with a single goal of exploring a relationship issue, but as they open up and progress through the process, they might feel the need to explore their sense of mortality and their fear concerning that. Therefore, flexibility will be required for the therapist to foster the client's sense of autonomy and respond to any change to goals communicated by the client.

In the initial assessment, Anne identified her goal as "I want to feel like me again" (Fleet, 2019, p. 115). She perceived her life and her self-image as changed for the worse since her accident. The compound fracture to her femur had resulted in many losses, including her dancing. However, as the therapy progressed, she became more self-accepting of her losses and limitations, realising that she could not be as physically able as before her accident. Her goal changed to finding something new, which would give her meaning and a purpose in life, and she represented this with an object of a key, which she placed in the sand and stated, "*that key … it spurred me on to find something else … do you know what I mean*"? (Fleet, 2019, p. 118).

Another aspect of the initial assessment concerns the case formulation stage. Cooper and Dryden (2016) advocate being creative during this stage with the client, and they refer to a structured shared activity using a timeline map. They suggest that the therapist holds the pen unless the client prefers to do so, and the exercise involves drawing a timeline. First, "*0 Years*" is written on the left of the line and *"now"* further along, representing the client's current situation of why they are seeking counselling, leaving some space on the right for future hopes. The client begins talking about their current issue whilst the therapist locates this on the timeline in the "now" position.

The client is helped to reflect on their lives and identifies significant issues in their past, each located at the specific age it occurred. The therapist can then facilitate a conversation to make any possible links from the client's past experience to their current distress.

An example of this could be if the client were currently experiencing panic attacks during public speaking, and in their past, as a child, they were heavily criticised for poor communication and may now see a link between the two experiences. A further example could be if the client is currently experiencing low mood after being made redundant, and in their past, they experienced a bereavement but were unable to grieve for some reason. A possible link may be that their current loss has triggered unresolved grief from their past loss to emerge, exasperating their current distress.

Worden (1991) suggested that a loss not sufficiently grieved for might be hidden and triggered by a future loss. The grieving of both losses can result in excessive grieving and possibly conditions such as depression. Worden (1991) discussed how delayed grief reactions could be inked to insufficient social support at the time of loss. He gave the example of a pregnant woman whose children died in an accident, and she was informed not to get too distressed, as this may be a risk to her unborn child. Taibbi (2017). (www.psychologytoday. com/gb/blog/fixing-families/201706/six-signs-incomplete-grief   Retrieved January 2021) also suggested that a person who has incomplete grief does not go through the natural healing process, resulting in emotional disturbance and persistent low-grade depression.

Once the timeline is complete, the therapist may ask the client whether they think their past loss has any possible link to their low mood now, but it is essential to stay close to their perceptions without making assumptions. At the end of the session, there needs to be sufficient time for reflection between the client and the therapist. When it is a shared collaborative active process, case formulation can increase understanding of the possible reasons why the client is currently experiencing distress and can identify several goals and ways of working in therapy (Cooper & Dryden, 2016).

Following the case formulation stage, the client and the therapist can work collaboratively, deciding how they will work together in therapy by setting the tasks and methods, with the therapist asking purposeful questions – for example, asking an anxious client, "What do you think might help you work on you becoming less anxious"? or "How have you managed your anxiety in the past"? As well as establishing a collaborative encounter and developing understanding, this dialogical process can contribute to the client feeling valued. It becomes apparent that they have an essential part to play in the therapy, and this realisation can avoid establishing a power imbalance with the therapist becoming dominant and deciding what direction the therapy should take.

Cooper and Dryden (2016), who view the client "as a co-participant in therapy" (p. 19), suggest how clients often have their own ideas about what helped them in the past and beliefs about what might help them now. However, therapist transparency is an essential feature in pluralistic therapy, with the sharing of the therapist's ideas and knowledge, drawing on other theoretical perspectives and practices on what might help the client (Cooper & Dryden, 2016). For example, the therapist may draw upon cognitive behavioural therapy by suggesting a breathing technique that could be facilitated at the end of the first session to help an anxious client, which they can use outside therapy. It is crucial to facilitate the client to be engaged in any decision-making about the tasks and methods so that the relationship is collaborative from the first meeting.

Sand-tray sessions

First session

When beginning the first session, the therapist can remind the client of their goal/s and how they agreed to work together.

Shirley (Fleet, 2019) identified two goals: first, wanting to manage her anxiety, and the second, to say aloud a difficult thing she had not said before. Together we agreed to include a relaxation technique at the end of the first session, so Shirley was reminded of this and wanted to go ahead. The breathing exercise incorporated colour. Shirley chose the colours red for breathing out her anxiety and blue for breathing in calm energy, which she repeated until her anxiety subsided. The exercise facilitated at the end of the session, followed by a discussion with Shirley on how she could plan to use this between sessions when she became aware of her anxiety building. She found this helpful and continued to do this throughout the time she was receiving therapy. McLeod (2018) would support this strategy and argued that the therapist could engage in "instructional psycho-educational talk" when suggesting a pluralistic counselling task.

When beginning the session, the client is invited to sit in front of the sand tray, with the therapist sitting at the side. It is helpful to remind the client how the objects can help them explore their thoughts and feelings by saying something like, "So the objects act as physical symbols to represent your experience, which can help you work through what you came here to talk about." It might also help if you ask the client whether they have any questions. Once the client is happy to go ahead a simple direction of:

> So when you are ready, search through the objects, and whichever jump out at you, pick them up and place them in the basket. You can choose

as few or as many as you want to and go back and select more during the session. You can work with dry sand or add water if you want to mould the sand into hills, for example. There is no rush, take all the time you need.

Usually, clients will bring the objects over to the sand tray and sit down when ready to progress. Some will begin by placing them in the sand without direction; others will need a prompt from the therapist such as "so when you are ready, begin placing them in the sand." At this time, it is usually best for the therapist to remain quiet and watch as the client creates a sand display. It is common for a client to either sit back in the chair or look at the therapist once their initial display is complete. The therapist can then state, "so when you are ready, begin talking about the objects. Whatever thoughts and feelings come to mind, feel free to express them."

Often, clients will select a first object that holds some significance for them and will commonly place this in the centre of the sand tray. For example, Anne (Fleet, 2019) immediately selected the object of a woman sitting in a wheelchair and placed it in the centre of the sand. This powerful symbol had an immediate impact as Anne became emotional and expressed her fear of the possibility that she may be unable to walk in the future due to her accident. During this process, it was essential to stay with and support Anne but without intervening too much. It might be appropriate to tentatively ask whether the client is okay to continue, and Anne responded to this question with a simple nod. Once Anne had stopped crying and became calmer, she began to place other objects in the sand, exploring other experiences such as her personal relationships. At the end of this session, Anne shared how she needed a good cry; it is crucial that the therapist does not rush in and rescue the client from their emotional expression.

Ruth (Fleet, 2019) selected an object of a demon monster almost immediately, placing it in the centre of the sand tray and stating, "that's my mother, *she said she didn't love me … I was a kid … she had a cane that she used to hit me with … I want to smash it!*" (Fleet, 2019, p. 185). Like Anne, this first object held huge significance for Ruth. It symbolised the physical and psychological abuse she experienced as a child by her mother. Ruth went on to express her anger and explored her abusive past for most of the first session. Although her initial goal was to make changes regarding having a romantic relationship with a man, it was her historical abuse that she needed to explore in this session. Once again, this indicated the necessity to take a flexible approach regarding the client's goals, aiming to stay alongside them in the sessions.

During the following sessions, Ruth did focus on her relationship issue with men but still valued the first session when she explored her abuse. At the end of therapy, she stated, "I have talked about things that I have hidden for a long time. It has felt good to open up" (Fleet, 2019, p. 246).

At the end of this first session, it is helpful to have some time to reflect on how the client thought the session went and to take photographs. When taking photographs and tidying away the objects, these can be decided between therapist and client. Some clients will want to tidy the objects away themselves; others will ask the therapist to do it when they have left the room. In my experience, most clients like to be present when photographs are taken and given the option to have a copy.

Continuing sessions

The second and subsequent sand-tray sessions will be collaborative, where purposeful dialogue is built into the process between therapist and client. For example, a subsequent session could begin with the client exploring how they have been since the previous session, or they may come with an idea of what they want to focus on and confidently begin to select objects. Other clients may ask to see the photograph from the first session to help give them some focus and link the current session to the last. Alternatively, they might not know where to begin and seek guidance from the therapist. Whatever the focus, it will be essential to stay alongside the client and respond to a request by them, helping them become familiar with the process, fostering their autonomy.

The therapist in pluralistic sand-tray therapy will adopt a fluent role; at times, they will be the empathic listener, offering the core conditions (Rogers, 1957), reflecting the client's thoughts and feelings, and making empathic paraphrases of the client's speech. At other times, they will take on the role of co-director by asking questions, making suggestions, and offering challenges; as the client places the objects in the sand, which serves as a stage for them to act out their experience in a type of metaphorical experiential theatre (Fleet, 2019).

In the fourth session, Anne (Fleet, 2019) disclosed how she could have temper tantrums and laughed as she described this. At this point, the question was put to her if she could select an object to represent this tendency, and Anne readily accepted this challenge, placing an object of a young girl, laying it face down in the sand.

Anne explored her life as the youngest of the family, how spoilt she was, describing her temper tantrums as not stopping until she got what she wanted from her mother, describing herself as a "spoilt brat." Anne reflected on this aspect of self and began to make links from her tantrums in childhood to the tantrums she has as an adult when trying to get her way with her husband. After exploring this for some time, she concluded how she needed to change, aiming to be kinder to her husband when she could not get her way.

Another link Anne made regarding this tendency was to her accident. Her "spoilt child" was angry, she wanted to have her old leg back, but further along in therapy, Anne began to accept that it would be impossible to get her way this time and reiterated her need to change. Her accident had been too severe; she would always have limitations regarding what she could do physically. Although this was a painful process for Anne, in the end of session feedback, Anne stated, "Good session ... made me realise how I still can have those temper tantrums" (Fleet, 2019. p. 243).

This suggestion made to Anne of representing her temper tantrum behaviour with an object helped her engage in "metacommunication." McLeod (2018) stated how purposeful questioning involved "metacommunication" described as "the act of standing back from the on-going flow of conversation, reflecting on (or inviting reflection on) the intentions and/or reactions of the speaker and/or listener" (p. 83). Anne began to reflect on her life as a spoilt child and symbolised this aspect by laying a small child face down in the sand. Her "spoilt brat" aspect presented onto the "stage" of the "experiential theatre" (the sand tray) facilitated her to explore her phenomenological experience, helping her make links to her current behaviour.

Purposeful questioning facilitates the client to reflect in a deep and meaningful way; it can also help them work on "edge of awareness" (Gendlin, 1996) material and facilitate unconscious processing (Eimers, 2014). Eimers (2014) referred to a case study and described how the client's "unconscious was unravelling a very complex problem" (p. 136) when engaged in sand-tray therapy. Pearson and Wilson (2009) described how many causes of psychological and emotional disturbance negatively impact a person's life, originating in the past, which may not be in conscious awareness. The outcome of "edge of awareness" and unconscious processing in therapy often results in the client gaining insight, and this new understanding can be a healing experience.

The therapist will need to listen and watch out for discrepancies or repetitive behaviour that may block or restrict the therapeutic process. For example, a client may place an object in the corner of the sand tray in different sessions but avoid any reference to it, indicating a reluctance to talk about a significant issue. This behaviour can be challenged by the therapist and may involve a congruent statement such as "I notice you have placed X in the corner again, I'm wondering what that represents for you"? Alternatively, the therapist may believe that a more substantial challenge may be more helpful. For example, they could suggest that the object be placed in the centre of the sand tray. This position makes it more difficult for the client to ignore the experience symbolised by the object and is a concrete invitation to work beyond their defences.

Another behaviour that can help a client explore further is when the client works with the sand, such as smoothing, digging, or burying objects. Using the sensory experiences of touch can facilitate the therapeutic process, bringing change (Hass-Cohen, 2008), and Montague (1986) described how touch completes the experience, adding the missing dimension to the client's process. To facilitate purposeful discussion, a simple reflection of "... and you've buried the object" or "you are smoothing the sand" can be made. Depending on the client's response, exploratory questions could help them explore further.

A helpful aspect of the therapeutic process is to have some form of mid-therapy feedback. Feedback can be verbal, written, or a combination of the two, and purposeful conversations can help the client get the most they can out of therapy, helping them achieve their goals. It is vital to establish a "culture of feedback" (Cooper & McLeod, 2011, p. 129) so both the client and the therapist can make any necessary changes.

Required changes will depend on the individual client having the therapy, but examples of what they want the therapist to do may include, "helping me focus on my feelings more" or "for you to be more challenging." Dallos and Vetere (2005) argued that a "feedback loop," with the counsellor adjusting their actions in response to client feedback, is necessary to demonstrate, respect, and enhance client agency. McLeod (2018) is in agreement and stated how engaging in feedback conversations will help the client to gain "a greater sense of agency and purpose in relation to their process of recovery …" (p. 104). For the relationship to be openly collaborative, there needs to be space for these purposeful conversations to occur during therapy and in the end session.

Final session

In order to complete the final assessment and feedback process, it may be helpful to expand the time of the final session to 1.5 hours, with the last 30 minutes dedicated to completing the post-therapy questionnaire and collecting feedback from the client. In my experience, most clients will be aware that this is the final session and often are in a reflective frame of mind, many looking back over their experience of engaging in sand-tray therapy. For example, in her last session, Ruth (Fleet, 2019) placed a piece of rail-track in the sand, positioning a knotted ball of string and a small coconut on the left and a silver butterfly on the right side. Ruth discussed how the structures on the left-hand side corresponded to her past abuse, and the butterfly on the right was how she felt at the end of therapy. She described how she had changed, *"I feel … bright … sparkling and stuff … and different with everybody else as well"* (Fleet, 2019, p. 132).

It is common for clients to symbolise their progress by selecting an object that represents how they see they have changed due to therapy. This representation can give an excellent anchor to begin discussing their experience of pluralistic sand-tray therapy. Completing the outcome measure, which maps change in the client's psychological well-being, is also a requirement in this last session. Examples of this type of questionnaire include CORE (Twigg & McInnes, 2010), The Patient Health Questionnaire (PHQ-9), and GAD-7Anxiety Severity (Spitzer et al., (2006) www.goodmedicine.org.uk Retrieved February 2020). However, a wide range of tools is available for use, and the outcome measure chosen will depend on the therapist's preference or the organisation they work for. A post-therapy outcome measure will be compared to the pre-therapy measure completed in the initial assessment. In pluralistic therapy, a purposeful discussion between therapist and client will focus on any improvement or not in the client's level of distress. Following this, a process measure concerned with gaining feedback on the client's experience of therapy will be carried out. As with outcome measures, there is a variety available to measure the therapeutic relationship's various dimensions, such as the Alliance Negotiation Scale (Doran et al., 2012). This scale measures the degree of collaboration between client and therapist.

Qualitative reflections are also a helpful way to collect feedback that enables a client to share their view of the usefulness of therapy. This type of feedback can be done either verbally or written down, and because the client describes their feedback in their own words, it is conducive to dialogical conversation. The following examples come from the case study (Fleet, 2019) and cover written end of session and end of therapy client feedback. In her feedback at the end of session one, Grace stated, "*I was able to express my feelings … it gives a visual focus as well as talking*" (Fleet, 2019, p. 247). This feedback gave some insight into how the session had helped Grace to express her feelings and demonstrated how she valued the visual sand display, in addition to talking.

Ruth wrote how she had worked in session three, stating, "*Took a look into what my feelings from the past mean … I'm getting to grips with them*" (p. 246). In her end of therapy feedback, she wrote, "*Helped me talk about things from my past*" (p. 246). In the final feedback, Ruth encapsulated how she had achieved closure, "*… put that to bed now*" (p. 246). This comment indicated how she perceived herself as moving from getting to grips with her feelings in session three to her closure at the end of therapy, indicating progression.

Jackie shared her views at the end of session four on how the presence of the symbolic object and I, as her therapist, was helping her explore and express her feelings, "*With you probing in the right areas helped me go deeper and to go with my feelings. The object being in front of you … which you can't ignore*" (Fleet, 2019, p. 245).

John arrived for his first session describing how he was feeling numb and could not cry. However, during the session, he wept, and at the end of this first session, he was relieved, stating, "*It's all about trying to let it all out*". However, at the end of session four, John remained sitting in the chair. He had worked on his anger towards a tutor whom he had a difficult altercation with concerning an assignment. He still felt angry at the end of the session and did not want to leave feeling like this.

I suggested I could talk him through a relaxation technique, either breathing or visualisation, which he gave some consideration. He decided he would like a breathing exercise, and as this was facilitated, his body language began to change, his shoulders dropped, and he sat back in his chair, looking much calmer. John then completed the end of session feedback stating, "*Felt angry today but glad you help me relax at the end*" (Fleet, 2019, p. 244).

Anne's end of session feedback in session one focused on her cathartic experience related to her fear of the possibility that she may not be able to walk due to her severe accident. Her comment on the session was, "*It was hard, but I had to let it out ... not sure ... hope it helps*".

Anne shared how she knew she had to express her pain but still questioned whether the sand-tray therapy would be helpful. However, at the end of the second session, her perception changed to now perceiving that the therapy was beneficial, "*Initially I did not know how it would help, but after this session, it felt it to be very beneficial*" (Fleet, 2019, p. 243).

At the end of therapy, Shirley communicated that she had met her goals of managing her panic attacks and saying something aloud she had not spoken of before. She revisited both of those goals and shared how the sessions had helped her. Shirley stated, "*Helped me talk about my panic*" and "*it gave me the chance to explore things in my life which I initially had problems talking about*" (Fleet, 2019, p. 242). She had managed to speak the unspoken as she questioned whether God was real. Shirley was able to voice the unspoken to someone who was not going to judge her, bringing a phenomenological shift; she experienced a sense of relief and validated her questioning of religion, which she had been taught throughout her life was taboo.

The end of session and end of therapy qualitative feedback can be vital for the therapist to acknowledge what is working well and what needs to be improved.

Qualitative feedback, combined with outcome measures and process measures, gives a more thorough understanding of the efficacy of therapy. Loewenthal (2013) adopted a creative approach of working with pictures with adolescents where the client's final pictures indicated their progression.

Loewenthal (2013) stated how a final picture in this type of therapy has the "potential evaluation of therapeutic change may be a beneficial and complementary, if not alternative, approach to evaluation approaches such as GAD-7, PHQ-9 and CORE-10" (p. 31). One client Winston (pseudonym) chose a picture of a pack of cards representing him not finding the right words to express his experience previously. However, at the end of therapy, Loewenthal described how Winston's evaluation scores increased, and the final picture selected was interpreted as him finding his "voice and moving forward" (p. 31), now being able to express his concerns. This final picture in Loewenthal's approach is similar to the final sand display in pluralistic sand-tray therapy, as often the client will select an object to represent their progress and how they have changed as a result of therapy.

However, collecting any type of feedback needs to be a collaborative process and consider the client's preference. Some clients will be happy to complete various forms of feedback, whilst others may only want to give verbal feedback, so it is essential to respect their agency.

References

Churchill, W. (1874–1965). www.goodreads.com Retrieved 12 April 2021.

Cooper, M., & Dryden, W. (Eds.) (2016). *Handbook of pluralistic counselling and psychotherapy*. London: Sage.

Cooper, M., & McLeod, J. (2011). *Pluralistic counselling and psychotherapy*. London: Sage.

Dallos, R., & Vetere, A. (2005). *Researching psychotherapy and counselling*. Berkshire: Open University Press.

Doran, J. M., Safran, J. D., Waizmann, V., Bolger, K., & Muran, C. (2012). Alliance Negotiation Scale. *Psychotherapy Research*, *22*(6), 710–719.

Eimers, A. (2014). Preparing for death: A child's experience. *Journal of Sandplay Therapy*, *23*(1), 135–144.

Fleet, D. (2019). *Transformation hidden in the sand: Developing a theoretical framework using a sand-tray intervention with adult clients*. Doctoral thesis. Staffordshire University. Stoke-on-Trent. Available from Ethos STORE – Staffordshire Online Repository. https://eprints.staffs.ac.uk/id/eprint/5763

Gendlin, E. T. (1996). *Focusing orientated psychotherapy*. New York: Guildford Press.

Hass-Cohen, N. (2008). CREATE: Art Therapy Relational Neuroscience Principles (ATR-N). In N. Hass-Cohen & R. Carr (Eds.), *Art therapy and clinical neuroscience*. London: Jessica Kingsley Publishers.

Loewenthal, D. (2013). Talking pictures therapy as brief therapy in a school setting. *Journal of Creativity in Mental Health*, *8*, 21–34.

McLeod, J. (2018). *Pluralistic therapy: Distinctive features*. London: Routledge, Taylor & Francis Group.

Montague, A. (1986). *Touching: The human significance of the skin*. London: HarperCollins.

O'Neill, S. (1999). Social work – a profession? *Journal of Social Work Practice*, *13*(1), 9–18. doi: 10.1080/026505399103467.

Pearson, M., & Wilson, H. (2009). *Using expressive arts to work with mind, body and emotions: Theory and Practice*. London: Jessica Kingsley Publishers.

Rogers, C. R. (1957). The necessary and sufficient conditions of therapeutic personality change. *Journal of Consulting Psychology*, *21*, 95–103.

Spitzer, R. L., Williams, J. W. W., & Kroenke, K. et al. (2006). The Patient Health Questionnaire (PHQ-9) and GAD-7Anxiety Severity (All PRIME-MD and PHQ materials were developed, with an educational grant from Pfizer Inc. (www.goodmedicine.org.uk Retrieved February 2020).

Taibbi, R. (2017). Six signs of incomplete grief. *Psychology Today*. (www.psychologytoday.com/gb/blog/fixing-families/201706/six-signs-incomplete-grief Retrieved January 2021).

Twigg, E., & McInnes, B. (2010). *YP-CORE user manual*, Version 1.0, CORE. Rugby: Information Management Systems Ltd.

Worden, J. W. (1991). *Grief counselling and grief therapy. A handbook for the mental health practitioner* (3rd ed.). Hove: Brunner-Routledge.

Chapter 9

Pluralistic sand-tray therapy and specific client issues

The boisterous sea of liberty is never without a wave
(Thomas Jefferson [1743–1826] https://founders.archives.gov)

A client who comes to therapy wanting to be free of their overwhelming psychological distress is likely to face a challenging journey. However, taking the first step to come to therapy, often, which they do under their own steam, might be the most challenging step they will take. From then on, there will be two, the client and the therapist, working together to overcome further challenges to master the client's distress.

A therapist is likely to work with a wide range of issues when counselling clients. However, there are some issues that the therapist is faced with regularly, including anxiety, depression, loss, guilt and shame, relationship problems, suicidal thoughts, and self-harm.

This chapter will explore each of these presenting issues and explore how pluralistic sand-tray therapy takes a collaborative approach when working with that particular issue.

Anxiety

"Anxiety is one of the most distressing emotions that people feel" (Greenberger & Padesky, 1995, p. 174). Greenberger and Padesky (1995) describe how anxiety depicts several problems, with most people being aware of the physical symptoms.

The physical symptoms can include "jitteriness, tension, sweaty palms, light-headedness, difficulty breathing, increased heart rate and flushed cheeks" (Greenberger & Padesky, 1995, p. 174). In addition, common distorted thoughts linked to anxiety begin with "what if …"?, with the individual perceiving they are in danger, feeling threatened, or feeling vulnerable (Greenberger & Padesky, 1995).

Panic, described as acute anxiety or fear, has a "combination of distinct emotions and physical symptoms" (Greenberger & Padesky, 1995, p. 182).

DOI: 10.4324/9781003158707-9

The physical symptoms are synonymous with those experienced with anxiety, but panic can also be associated with disorientation and catastrophic thoughts; often, the person perceives they are having a heart attack and are about to die (Greenberger & Padesky, 1995).

Some people will develop more severe and prolonged anxiety that could manifest into a disorder. The World Health Organization (WHO) defines anxiety disorders arising "in a number of forms including phobic, social, obsessive-compulsive (OCD), post-traumatic disorder (PTSD) or generalised anxiety disorders" (Ritchie & Roser, 2018 https://ourworldindata.org/mental-health Retrieved February 2021).

The WHO estimated that 284 million people worldwide had an anxiety disorder in 2017, suffering moderate to severe symptoms (Ritchie & Roser, 2018).

Abbing et al. (2019) argued that non-verbal art therapy, which involves drawing, painting, sculpting, and clay modelling, "is considered to be suitable for individuals with anxiety" (https://doi.org/10.1155/2019/4875381 Retrieved 12 March 2021).

Abbing suggested that this therapy is beneficial for clients who struggle to identify and express their feelings or use rationalising as a coping mechanism. This argument is based on the rationale that a client talking about their anxiety could evoke fear; however, with non-verbal art therapy, verbal communication during the artwork is avoided. In addition, the distance when producing the art can bring a sense of control, contributing to the client being able to manage their anxious emotions more effectively (Abbing et al, 2019).

Although verbal communication is a central feature of sand-tray therapy, distancing is also relevant; the client forms a physical picture of their anxiety in the sand, helping them take the observer–experiencer position. This perspective enables them to avoid becoming overwhelmed (Fleet, 2019), and the distance helps them stay with the process, exploring their phenomenological experience, which for an anxious client is likely to include fear underpinning their anxiety.

When setting goals, tasks, and methods with an anxious client, the therapist needs to consider helping the client manage their anxiety or panic outside of therapy in addition to how they will work together in therapy sessions. A relaxation technique is one approach that can help the client between sessions. However, the choice will be a collaborative decision, with the client stating their preference for either a controlled breathing technique or a visualisation (Chapter 2). It is a good idea to facilitate the technique at the end of the first session to familiarise the client with the process. At the beginning of the next session, it is helpful to have a dialogical conversation on how this has gone. Any changes that might be required can then be agreed upon for practising the technique the following week.

In the initial assessment, anxious clients will often say they do not want to feel anxious or be able to manage their anxiety or panic. Dryden (Cooper & Dryden, 2016) suggested that anxious clients usually focus on their feelings and a discussion concerning healthy anxiety when facing a threat can be helpful. Reaching a state of healthy anxiety is more likely to be achieved than eradicating anxious feelings completely. Dryden (Cooper & Dryden, 2016) described this as functional anxiety compared to problematic anxiety, which results in the client experiencing distress. This type of discussion can help clients set a more realistic goal of reducing their anxiety so that they do not become overwhelmed daily.

When deciding tasks, Dryden (Cooper & Dryden, 2016) discussed how he would invite an anxious client "to consider the idea of anxiety as a plant" (pp. 188–189). This metaphor exercise begins by Dryden asking "what conditions would lead to your anxiety to thrive and what conditions would lead your anxiety to wither in the long-term" (2016, p. 188). This exercise helps the client identify specific behaviour and distorted thinking that maintain their level of anxiety. Also, it may indicate changes that are needed to reduce the level of anxiety the client is experiencing. For example, a condition on the thriving list may be "catastrophic thoughts," adapted to "realistic thinking" on the wither list (Cooper & Dryden, 2016). Dryden (Cooper & Dryden, 2016) also discussed how it is essential to identify the client's strengths when setting tasks. For example, a strength could be that the client is good at trying out new things and is willing to try a different behaviour when their anxiety begins to build. However, this will be unique to each client, so a dialogical conversation is required to meet each client's needs.

There is a range of therapy methods, from the broad to the specific; in pluralistic sand-tray therapy, the way of working is decided collaboratively between the client and the therapist. When clients select an object to represent their anxiety, some will choose a monster or a demon, whilst others choose an animal or a reptile they see as threatening; however, others may choose a more abstract object such as a tangled ball of string or a large gnarled stone.

In my practice, clients have sometimes used a small skull to represent their anxiety, frequently symbolising their fear of death. Whatever the object chosen, the therapist needs to stay close to the client's meaning and help them voice their fear. The client can then focus on the object representing their fear without becoming overwhelmed. It is as if they have taken one step away from their fear without losing connection to it, and they begin exploring their inner world perceptions and hopefully achieve a phenomenological shift by the end of therapy.

When a client is preoccupied with their fear and unable to make a shift, it can help to suggest that they select a protective object (Chapter 5). This object is a symbol of strength and a metaphor for protection. Common protective objects include spiritual symbols such as an angel or the Buddha, or a power animal, like a lion or a tiger, often placed next to the anxiety object in the sand, bringing a sense of relief and perceived protection for the client.

I have often witnessed a client act out the destruction of the anxiety object by either knocking it over with the protective object or burying it in the sand.

This action can bring a shift in the client's thinking, and some have used this power object in a guided visualisation facilitated in therapy. Other clients have also visualised this protective object in their mind's eye during the week when they begin to feel anxious, giving them a sense of protection against the underpinning fear. Some have purchased an ornament or painting of their protective object and placed it in their home, giving them a continued sense of peace and protection. However, most clients will request a photograph of this object in the sand to take home, reminding them of the protective symbolism.

Depression

McLeod discussed how a diagnostic view of depression would describe it as "a combination of symptoms that reflect different aspects of life, for example, low mood, guilt, self-critical thoughts, sleep and appetite disturbance and social isolation" (McLeod, In Cooper & Dryden, 2016, p. 174). Globally, "over 300 million people are estimated to suffer from depression, equivalent to 4.4% of the world's population" (World Health Organization, 2017, p. 5. https://apps.who.int/iris/bitstream/handle/10665/254610/WHO-MSD-MER-2017.2-eng.pdf?sequence=1&isAllowed=y).

As with anxiety, the problem may become severe, with some people developing a depressive disorder. A disorder is diagnosed when the depression is long-lasting, is recurrent, and interferes with the individual's way of life, impairing their ability to function in the world. The WHO defines depressive disorders as "characterized by sadness, loss of interest or pleasure, feelings of guilt or low self-worth, disturbed sleep or appetite, feelings of tiredness, and poor concentration" (WHO, 2017, p. 7. https://apps.who.int/iris/bitstr eam/handle/10665/254610/WHO-MSD-MER-2017.2-eng.pdf?sequence= 1&isAllowed=y), stating that if depression is acutely severe, it can lead to suicide.

Greenberger and Padesky (1995) argued that depression includes sad mood and other cognitive, emotional, physical, and behavioural symptoms and, when severe, can interfere with an individual's life experience. For example, Beck (1967) linked negative thinking to depression, such as self-criticism and general negativity about the world and the future (Greenberger & Padesky, 1995). Depressed people tend to "remember negative aspects of their experiences more readily than positive or neutral aspects." (Greenberger & Padesky, 1995, p. 161).

McLeod described how the multiple causes and treatments for depression are conducive to pluralistic therapy, with its flexible and collaborative stance. It also draws on the strengths of other approaches and considers the client's perception of their depression (McLeod, In Cooper & Dryden, 2016). Depression is a complex phenomenon, and understanding the client's view and setting goals will help establish how the therapy will proceed, and successful therapy is likely to foster change to their cognitive, emotional, physical, and behavioural experience.

McLeod (In Cooper & Dryden, 2016) stated how "some depressed people may present themselves as passive, defeated and too stuck to care" (p. 180). When working with a depressed client, a lack of motivation to engage in the therapy can be common. In this circumstance, a more collaborative, directive approach by the therapist using structured sand-tray sessions can help the client who wants or needs direction before engaging. The following structured sessions might be helpful.

Transforming a client's present depressive state into a positive future-orientated attitude

McLeod (In Cooper & Dryden, 2016) discussed how a depressed client could transform their depressed state by focusing on "how they would like their life to be at some point in the future" (p. 179). Commonly, depressed clients will ruminate about their inadequacies based on negative past experience (McLeod, In Cooper & Dryden, 2016).

A structured sand-tray session can begin by exploring what, if anything, brings the client pleasure. A client can be guided to create a sand display by selecting objects to represent how they would like their life to be in the future. The client is facilitated to express their thoughts and feelings related to the picture in the sand, then is helped to identify how they could bring change to experience some pleasure in everyday life.

When even partially integrated into their life, the client is likely to experience a phenomenological shift in their inner perceptions. If this change, no matter how small, can be repeated each day, it could result in a more positive future orientation for the client. Also, there might be positive changes regarding their behaviour and improvements in their relationships.

Adopting a four focus approach with depression

This structured session focuses on four areas: the client's thoughts, feelings, physical symptoms, and behaviour relating to their depression. The therapist could suggest that the client split the sand tray into four sections (thoughts, feelings, physical symptoms, behaviour) and represent each of the four with objects relating to their depression. Once the client has explored each of these areas, the next step is to consider a manageable change. For distorted thinking, this might include seeking contradictions to negative thoughts, exploring alternatives, challenging the distorted thinking, or identifying a positive affirmation to repeat daily.

A relaxation technique may change the physical symptoms experienced, and behaviour change may involve integrating some daily outdoor exercise. Concerning the associated feelings, the client would need help to identify and express these. If the client is numb and cannot connect to their feelings, the therapist could facilitate a creative visualisation to help them break through the resistance. However, sand-tray therapy's symbolic nature can help the client in this regard, as feelings tend to emerge due to its projective nature and touch process. New goals, represented by objects, could then be established at the end of this session when the client and the therapist reflect on the session.

The therapist might also draw on the solution-focused approach (SFT) (de Shazer et al., 1986). Taylor (2009) used sand tray and integrated this in her SFT, aiming to shift the attention away from the client's present problem and exploring "what the client is and isn't doing to address the problem" (Neimer In Cooper & Dryden, 2016, p. 226). Trepper et al. (2010) stated, "causes of problems may be extremely complex, their solutions do not necessarily need to be" (p. 1). Therefore, this approach is future-orientated and focuses on the solution and not on the client's problem.

This change in focus could be incorporated into a structured sand-tray session and suggest the client select objects to represent how their life would be if a change had already occurred, which may help them understand how their psychological state would be different. It might also provide the opportunity to help the client with their motivation by perceiving "a light at the end of the tunnel," signifying that they can recover and have a more positive future.

However, a therapist may believe that using this early in therapy ignores the underlying issue; this session could be incorporated towards the end of therapy once the client has already explored their thoughts and feelings concerning their distress. However, this will not be in line with SFT, which does not focus on the problem.

Mobilising the client's everyday resources

Cooper and McLeod (2011) discuss how cultural resources can help a client bring change, offer social connection, and be put to therapeutic use for the client. Such resources include reading, cooking, painting, spiritual practices, and outdoor activities (Cooper & McLeod, 2011). There is likely to be something in the client's past that gave them pleasure to explore in the session. Sometimes, a client has forgotten the positive feeling that those resources brought, and working with the symbolic objects can help them reflect on their past experience at a phenomenological level. Such reflection can remind the client how much pleasure and meaning they experienced in the past, helping build change by integrating a past activity into the present.

In my practice, I have worked with depressed clients who have taken up past activities such as writing poetry, painting, playing the guitar, golf, running, cycling, going back to the gym, or becoming a member of their church again, which helped them regain some of the pleasure and social connection they had lost during their depression. Re-establishing a past resource can be an essential element to the client's progress regarding their depression. However, each client is unique and will perceive their depression in their own way, and if the therapist communicates an expectation that the client "should" take up an activity, it may only serve to exacerbate the client's sense of failure if they feel they cannot or do not want to set this as a goal. Therefore, it is essential to work collaboratively, empathise with the client, and respect their autonomy and personal understanding without establishing an expectation of how to change their behaviour.

Helping establish congruent emotions within the client

A person who is depressed is likely to be either emotionally numb or experience diffuse (widespread) emotional pain (McLeod, In Cooper & Dryden, 2016). A client who cannot express their feelings might contribute to their depression, indicating a need for change to move towards self-regulation of emotion. McLeod (In Cooper & Dryden, 2016) discussed how self-regulation of emotion includes the ability to be aware of one's own feelings, to be able to distinguish between various emotions, to understand triggers to various emotions, and to be able to express one's emotions appropriately. Any or all of these aspects could be identified as tasks or goals for the client.

Working creatively using the sand tray is particularly conducive to helping a client achieve self-regulation of emotion, as the symbolic representation of experience helps the client connect to their feelings. The visual and tactile process of seeing and touching the objects and sand establishes a state involving physical sensation, emotion, and thinking.

My view related to my clinical experience is that it can be more helpful to have an unstructured approach when focusing clients on expressing their feelings. I find that enabling them to work in a free and uninterrupted way helps them connect to their feelings more readily, with the therapist only responding to a client's cues, whether verbally or non-verbally. For example, a client's eye contact may suggest that they need the therapist to contribute, even if it is a simple touch of a hand on their hand, indicating "I am hearing you and will stay alongside you as you begin to explore and express this difficult emotion." However, depressed clients may need a more structured approach to help them connect to their feelings, which will be decided in collaboration between them and their therapist.

Loss

Loss is a vast topic and incorporates many losses experienced by people. Examples include bereavement, divorce, redundancy, progressing through life stages (e.g., child to teenager, menopause), loss due to physical injury, life-changing illness, leaving school, and loss in a relationship due to imprisonment.

A person will experience a loss in their unique way; therefore, the therapist needs to avoid making assumptions about how the client will think, feel, or behave concerning their loss.

Bereavement

Bereavement is generally a distressing but common experience, as most people will experience the death or loss of someone they love at some time during their life. Individuals can experience a range of emotions during the grief process, including shock, numbness, anger, guilt, and sadness (Royal College of Psychiatrists, 2020 www.rcpsych.ac.uk/mental-health/problems-disorders/bereavement). However, not all individuals will experience all of those emotions and, if they do, not necessarily in that order.

Gillies and Neimeyer (2006) discussed how Victor Frankl (1962) stated, "people are driven by a psychological need to find or create a sense of meaning and purpose in their lives" (Gillies & Neimeyer, 2006, p. 31), relating this to bereavement. For an individual experiencing grief after a close bereavement, finding meaning associated with the loss can help them adapt to a changed world (Gillies & Neimeyer, 2006).

It is common for a bereaved individual to "experience missing, longing and yearning for the deceased" (Gillies & Neimeyer, 2006, p. 33). Parkes (1996) described how a bereaved person could also experience other emotions and behaviours such as intrusive thoughts, fear, hopelessness, intense sadness, and social withdrawal.

Ambiguous loss

Boss (2000) described ambiguous loss as that which occurs without closure or with the individual having no understanding of why the loss occurred. Ambiguous loss is likely to result in the person searching for answers that interfere with the grief process, creating a state of unresolved grief. Such loss can include termination of pregnancy, a close relative going missing, and infertility. Alzheimer's disease or dementia is also an example of ambiguous loss as the person affected is still alive, but there is decreasing cognitive functioning over time. Boss (2010) described how there are two types of ambiguous loss: physical and psychological. Physical loss occurs when there is some damage or illness to the physical body. For example, a person may have a body part amputated due to a severe accident or lose the use of a particular body part and grieve for that loss. Psychological loss occurs when the individual grieves for a loss related to the psychological mind (Boss, 2010).

Disenfranchised grief

Doka (1989) coined the term disenfranchised grief and described it as a loss not socially sanctioned. Aloi (2009) described disenfranchised grief as that which goes unacknowledged by society, and such loss includes losing a pet and the loss of a family home. Having to move out of the family home due to financial reasons or being evicted can be particularly disconcerting, and for a child, the enormity of the change, even to their physical environment, can be overwhelming; yet this grief, likened to an invisible loss, is not usually recognised by others.

Kubler-Ross (1969) suggested how loss that carries social stigma could result in disenfranchised grief. For example, the breakup of a secret relationship, such as an extramarital affair or the diagnosis of a sexually transmitted disease, can induce disenfranchised grief. If the person experiences social stigma, they could also experience shame or guilt, exacerbating their emotional and psychological state. Some forms of loss, such as bereavement, are more widely recognised, with the expectation that a person who has lost someone close will grieve, yet for disenfranchised grief, there might not be any acknowledgement from others. A person who has suffered a loss that others do not understand can also feel lonely, can be discouraged from talking about their loss, and can suffer alone and in silence.

Anticipatory loss

Lindemann (1944) first introduced the notion of anticipatory grief in his paper "Acute Grief." Aldrich (1974) defined this type of grief as "any grief occurring prior to a loss, as distinguished from the grief which occurs at or after a loss" (p. 4). This type of loss can be associated with a terminal illness, and both the individual who is dying and a close relative can experience it (National Cancer Institute. http://ncinagpur.in/).

Although the period before the death of a loved one known to be dying can be harrowing and difficult, there can be some positive aspects. Firstly, it can allow the individual to resolve issues with the dying person and gives the opportunity to say goodbye (National Cancer Institute. www.cancer. gov/about-cancer/advanced-cancer/caregivers/planning/bereavement-hp-pdq#section/all). In addition, Pine (1974) suggested that an individual experiencing anticipatory grief could work through their loss, making them more able to cope with their loved one's death, having resolved their grief before the death.

Some individuals, when bereaved, seek therapy to help them cope so that they have an empathic listener to hear their experience of loss and "help them find some means of negotiating a life whose terrain has been made alien by their bereavement" (Neimeyer, In Cooper & Dryden, 2016, p. 211). People experiencing grief due to bereavement often have many questions as they struggle to make sense of their loss.

Such questions may include, Why did they die? Why me? How can I get on with my life without them? How can I still hold on to my religious or spiritual beliefs? Therapy can help the person explore these questions, even if a concrete answer is not possible, and by helping the client explore, reflect, and express their pain, they may eventually move to a place of acceptance as they integrate their loss and rebuild their life.

As a bereaved person struggles to make sense of losing a loved one, they may engage in some creative process. For example, Davidson (2017) described how memorial tattooing is a type of creative practice, which bereaved people sometimes engage in and "function to communicate experiences and emotions which may be so intense as to defy spoken language alone" (p. 33). Likewise, Swann-Thomas et al. (2021) stated, "Individuals who have been etched with a memorial tattoo offer a very unique and enlightening perspective on the grieving process" (p. 11).

The tattoo picture may serve to engage others by validating their loss experience and as a way of beginning to explore their grief in therapy.

The client's tattoo can also be incorporated into pluralistic sand-tray therapy, with them guided to create a picture in the sand of what each aspect of the tattoo means, then exploring their thoughts and feelings represented by the symbolic objects.

It is common for the bereaved to feel the need to talk about the story of their loss, yet Neimeyer (In Cooper & Dryden, 2016) suggested, it is common for the painful details to be missing in their communication. Rynearson and Salloum (2011) advocate "restorative retelling" that involves the client repeating the story of the person's death several times to fill in those gaps. The therapist will help the client express their painful emotions during this process until the client can tell the whole story and integrate the death of their loved one in a meaningful way.

Pluralistic sand-tray therapy can integrate "restorative retelling" (Rynearson & Salloum, 2011); the client will create a sand display of the story of the person's death by using symbolic objects. This process can be ongoing over several sessions, and photographs of the sand display taken if the client wishes to refer to them.

As the story's missing aspects emerge, represented by the symbolic objects, the sand display will develop until the client perceives the story as complete.

The physical, symbolic picture in the sand helps the implicit aspects emerge as the client explores their phenomenological experience of their loss, projecting their inner experience onto the objects. By working at the "edge of awareness" (Gendlin, 1984) and using a significant object as a phenomenological anchor, they can then find their "right" words to communicate their more painful experience, making the implicit explicit (Fleet, 2019). Working creatively to explore and express their grief can benefit some clients as objects in the sand establish a distance. They take one step out of their pain to become the observer–experiencer and manage to stay with the process without becoming overwhelmed.

This unstructured approach will most likely be appropriate for a client experiencing disenfranchised grief, helping them explore their phenomenological experience and related emotions, such as sadness, loneliness, shame, and guilt. A tentative, compassionate, and empathic approach by the therapist will likely build trust, encouraging the client to become more transparent in their communication and express their feelings.

With anticipatory grief, the various tasks and methods may depend on what point in the grief process a client presents for therapy. For example, if the client attends therapy prior to the loved one's death, the sessions may focus more on preparing for the death, emotionally, psychologically, and cognitively. However, if the loved one has died, therapy may help the client express their emotions and aid the telling of their story surrounding their loved one's death. As the client moves through the therapy and can think about their future without the deceased, it may help by suggesting they create a sand display of what they hope their life could look like in a year, helping them explore those possibilities.

In the initial assessment with a bereaved person who has agreed to therapy, it might be that during a dialogical discussion between the therapist and the client, the specific tasks agreed on could focus on behaviour change or relaxation techniques and incorporated in addition to the therapy sessions. For some clients where the loss is recent, these strategies might not be appropriate as they may be very distressed, being too immersed in their grief to be able to focus. Nonetheless, for a person who comes to therapy sometime after their loss, these techniques may give additional help. Typical of the pluralistic approach, this will involve a collaborative process, as the client's input will be essential in deciding which strategy will suit them best.

However, for a bereaved client who has no understanding of their loss in the case of ambiguous loss or a severely distressed client, an unstructured approach might be the most appropriate option. For example, the client might place only one object in the sand representing the person who had died and express their emotion over their loss, and the therapist needs to offer compassion and empathy and stay alongside the client, going at their pace.

Alternatively, the client may present as numb, and again it is important not to rush the process but stay alongside them, gently offering compassion and empathy. Sometime later on in the therapeutic process, it can also help the client create a sand display of good memories the client had with the deceased or the client's perception of the good qualities the person who died had, recognising and acknowledging the life story of the deceased.

Guilt and shame

Brown (2006) defines *shame* as "an intensely painful feeling or experience of believing we are flawed and therefore unworthy of acceptance and belonging" (p. 45). In Brown's study, participants used terms such as devastating, excruciating, and rejected in their descriptions of shame (Brown, 2006). Sanderson (2006) suggested how shame is focused overwhelmingly on the self, and any "reparation in shame requires the entire transformation of the self" (p. 327). Tangney and Dearing (2002) argued how there are no universal shame triggers but shame being person- and context-specific.

Some writers perceive shame as synonymous with guilt. Greenberger and Padesky (1995) stated how "guilt and shame are closely connected emotions" (p. 197), describing how guilt is related to when rules have been violated, and shame is when an individual perceives they have done something wrong and are inadequate in some way.

However, several scholars distinguish between guilt and shame (Brown, 2006; Sanderson, 2006; Dearing et al., 2005; Fossum and Mason, 1986; Lewis, 1971). This view describes how a person may feel guilt when they behave in a flawed way, in contrast to shame due to the person viewing themself as flawed (Brown, 2006). Tangney and Dearing (2002) argued: "shame and guilt are distinct emotional experiences that differ substantially along cognitive, affective and motivational dimensions" (p. 24). Fossum and Mason (1986) stated, "While guilt is a painful feeling of regret and responsibility for one's actions, shame is a painful feeling about oneself as a person" (p. 5).

Some writers argued that there are different types of shame, depending on the intensity and the cause. Bradshaw (2005) and Graham (2014) described toxic shame as highly intense and debilitating and link it to child abuse and trauma, the individual often dissociating toxic shame until they can cope with it.

Secret shame, described by Gilligan (1997), is when the individual feels ashamed to be ashamed. This state might result in the person keeping their shame a secret, as exposing their shame to another would be too overwhelming, yet they may live in fear that others will expose their shame. Finally, Paulus et al. (2014) described vicarious shame as when an individual experiences shame on behalf of another individual and links this to neuroticism. For example, a son or a daughter could experience vicarious shame if their parent was imprisoned for committing a crime.

Whatever type of shame a client is experiencing, it can be highly challenging for a therapist to facilitate the client to expose and explore their shame as they can often find it difficult to hold eye contact with a therapist. However, in sand-tray therapy, the client can look at the sand display, project their shame onto the objects, and make eye contact only when ready to, giving them a sense of control. The processes of externalising their inner experience and projection can be beneficial to the therapeutic process. The therapist will need to take a tentative and empathic approach as the client shares their pain associated with shame. At this point, rushing in too soon or being too challenging can result in the client disengaging and closing down, resulting in a block to the therapeutic process.

Brown (2006) suggests that therapy is likely to focus on the client's emotions, thoughts, and behaviours related to their shame and the social aspects of feeling trapped, powerless, and isolated. Brown (2006) views empathy as key to helping clients overcome their shame and argued how the therapist would need to see the world as the client sees it. She refers to a metaphor of a petri dish, suggesting that shame only needs three elements to grow: silence, secrecy, and judgement (Brown, 2006), arguing that shame cannot thrive in a supportive environment where empathy exists.

Relationship problems

"Interpersonal relationship problems are frequently found to be the most common issues to be brought to counselling" (Barker In Cooper & Dryden, 2016, p. 198). Although there is a great deal of research on intimate relationship problems, clients bring difficulties in other relationships. For example, such interpersonal difficulties can exist between parent and child, siblings, friends, and work colleagues.

Relationship difficulties are wide-ranging, including the client feeling frustrated with the other person, not getting their needs met in the relationship, continuously blaming the other person, or not acknowledging their part in relationship conflict.

Intimate relationships

Boisvert et al. (2011) argued how in intimate relationships, the "most common problems were related to communication, emotional affection or distance, specific areas of the current relationship, and lack of physical affection or sex" (p. 362). Difficulties in communication between intimate partners were common in several research studies (Geiss & O'Leary, 1981; Levenson et al., 1993; Doss et al., 2004). Geiss and O'Leary (1981) stated that communication problems were the most damaging to intimate relationships and reported other issues, including a lack of loving feelings, power struggles, extramarital affairs, and having unrealistic expectations of the marriage. A therapist is likely to face common issues in intimate relationships that clients may bring to therapy; however, there will still be specific problems to that individual client and their relationship.

Parent and child relationships

Stavrianopoulos et al. (2015) describe how parents of adolescent children can experience problems in their relationships. An adolescent is likely to experience a process of change, with them adjusting to separation-individuation, trying to keep a connection to their parents whilst becoming more autonomous (Allen & Land, 1999). Such change can cause profound changes, sometimes causing conflict and distress in the parent–child relationship (Bucx & van Wel, 2008). For example, a parent may become frustrated with the adolescent son or daughter who is beginning to express more alternative views that can cause friction in the relationship and feelings of anger, hurt, or sadness.

Hasseldine (2020) discussed how mother and daughter relationships could sometimes be problematic. There is a societal expectation that mothers and daughters "should" be close, which can exacerbate any conflict they may be experiencing in their relationship. Hasseldine (2020) suggested that it is common for mothers and daughters to blame themselves for the problems in their relationship, and one or both may seek therapy.

Childers (2010) argued how "there is a generational difference in the father-son relationship" (p. 3) (https://digitalcommons.liberty.edu/honors/115) Retrieved 25 March 2022). Such difference can impact the quality of the relationship between fathers and sons.

Birditt et al. (2009) argued how the parent–child relationship is one of the most emotional and long-lasting relationships. Many parent–child relationships are caring and supportive, but difficulties can range from minor problems to severe conflict (Birditt et al., 2009). Fingerman (2001) suggested that relationships with daughters tend to be closer, be emotionally intense, and have more conflict.

Sibling relationships

Greif (2016) described how relationships between siblings could last longer than many other relationships, and older siblings most likely having to support ageing parents; therefore, cooperation between siblings is essential. However, there is likely to be disagreements and sometimes tension between siblings, especially when they hold different views and opinions. In addition, Greif (2016) suggested that adult siblings often do not understand another sibling's behaviour and often feel misunderstood by the other, leading to ambivalence.

Work relationships

Relationships at work can be warm and supportive and positively impact the individual's work experience. However, some relationships at work can be challenging and destructive, negatively impacting the individual's life.

Workplace bullying is a type of persistent behaviour that can be verbal, nonverbal, psychological, or physical, resulting in the bullied individual feeling humiliated (Rayner & Cooper, 2006). It can negatively impact an individual's self-esteem and mental health, and as Farrell and Geist-Martin (2005) suggested, stress is the most predominant health concern linked to workplace bullying. Furthermore, Yildirim and Yildirim (2007) suggested how bullying that severely impacts an individual can result in post-traumatic stress and even suicide.

When a client brings a relationship issue to pluralistic sand-tray therapy, it is essential to identify their goals and expectations for therapy and establish tasks and methods for working together. During the purposeful discussion, it will become apparent whether an unstructured approach to sand tray, a structured approach, or a combination of the two is the most appropriate method for that client.

The symbolic objects can represent themselves and the other person/s in the relationship, whilst other objects can signify the dynamic between them. The client will work through their issue by projecting onto the objects. For example, sometimes the client can act out a conversation or an argument that occurred in the relationship, and the action of speaking from the object representing them and then the object representing the other can give an alternative perspective. This activity can also give a sense that they have spoken and been heard by the therapist, which might bring a sense of relief.

Once the client has explored and expressed their thoughts and feelings concerning the problematic relationship, sometimes, if appropriate, it can help if the therapist invites them to shift their focus. This shift can involve asking challenging questions such as, "so how do you think the other person might see the relationship/problem"? This prompt can help clients explore their own input into the relationship and possibly help develop empathy for the other.

The spatial awareness of objects symbolising the relationship can communicate meaning for the client. For example, objects placed closed together might represent a close relationship. In contrast to this, objects placed apart in the sand tray may represent a distant or an antagonistic relationship. Further on in therapy, the position of the objects may change in that they become closer or further apart. Any change in the spatial picture as the therapy continues can indicate progression.

For example, such progression may indicate conflict being resolved or by the client deciding to end a relationship.

Suicidal thoughts

The WHO stated how suicide "accounted for 1.5% of all deaths worldwide, bringing it into the top 20 leading causes of death in 2015" (2017, p. 14 www. who.int/mental_health/management/depression/prevalence_global_health_ estimates/en/ Retrieved 24 February 2021). However, Gliatto and Rai (1999) described how most people who have suicidal thoughts do not engage in suicide attempts, although suicidal thoughts are still considered a risk factor.

The causes for suicide ideation are complex, although there are some similar links amongst people who have suicidal thoughts. For example, Fergusson et al. (2000) identified certain life events related to suicide ideation, including alcohol abuse, unemployment, chronic illness, death of a family member, and end of an intimate relationship.

Bridge et al. (2006) suggested how the link between mothers with depression and an increased risk of suicide behaviours in their offspring is well established. Furthermore, Hammerton et al. (2015) argued how "children exposed to chronic severe maternal depression symptoms across childhood are at considerably increased risk for suicidal ideation later in adolescence" (p. 390).

Reeves (2010) discussed how a suicidal client could present various challenges for the therapist with safeguarding a significant consideration, but managing risk must not detract from the therapeutic process. A pluralistic approach that adopts a collaborative and shared responsibility around risk could be helpful, as the client is active in any discussion and decision made (Reeves, 2010).

When considering reducing the potential for harm, it is essential to draw on the client's resources for self-support. Establishing an atmosphere of openness is likely to foster trust, with the client more likely to share thoughts and feelings, which they may not have shared with anyone else. Reeves (2015) discussed the need for therapists to openly discuss their client's suicidal thinking with them, which can communicate that it is acceptable to talk about such a taboo topic and indicate that the therapist has heard them.

The tasks and methods for therapy may involve drawing on Cognitive Behavioural Therapy (CBT), which can help change clients' patterns of thinking and behaviour concerning their self-harm. However, a different client might feel the need to tell their story to an impartial, empathic listener. When working with a suicidal client, a narrative approach (Michel & Valach, 2001) with the client's story as a core feature may be drawn upon when establishing the tasks for therapy. Reeves (2017) suggested how "a discursive based exploration" (p. 606) should be considered the primary approach when working with clients who self-harm so that they can gain an understanding of their suicidal behaviour.

Pluralistic sand-tray therapy with the therapist adopting a gentle, non-judgemental presence can give the client a sense of ownership. They select the objects representing the story of their suicidal thoughts, creating a picture in the sand that is in front of their eyes, and the symbolism explored can bring insight and understanding. If the client is intensely focused on the sand work, the therapist can remain quiet and observe. Once the client's body language changes, seeking input, the therapist can respond either verbally or nonverbally, such as a nod; even in silence, there can be communication and collaboration.

Intentional self-harm

Walsh (2008) defines *self-harm* as "Intentional self-effected, low lethality bodily harm of a socially unacceptable nature, performed to reduce psychological distress" (p. 4). Self-harm is a complex multi-professional issue (Turp, 1999) with various professions, including health care, psychology, psychiatry, counselling, and education, aiming to understand its cause and how best to work with it (Fleet & Mintz, 2012). This range of professions has produced contrasting opinions on why people engage in this behaviour and the most effective psychological intervention.

One difference concerns the contrasting views of client progression for a person who self-harms and accesses therapy (Fleet & Mintz, 2012). For example, Shaw and Shaw (2007) view cessation of self-harm by the client as progression, so the goal for therapy will likely be to stop the behaviour. Similarly, Laye-Gindhu and Schonert-Reichl (2005) perceive self-harm as a maladaptive coping mechanism and view progression as replacing this behaviour with a more constructive alternative. In contrast, Spandler and Warner (2007) describe how Pembroke (1996) understands self-harm to be a legitimate coping mechanism and a therapist having the expectation that a client will stop can exacerbate the self-harm, arguing that "total cessation is not the only measure of progress; if we do less damage, take better care of ourselves, or feel better about ourselves, that can constitute progress too" (p. 166).

Gardner (2001) recognises the client gaining insight into why they self-harm as a step in progression. Furthermore, Andover et al. (2005) suggested that clients who begin to talk about and express their feelings concerning their self-harm contribute to their recovery. These different perspectives on client progression highlight the debates around self-harm (Fleet & Mintz, 2012).

Taking a pluralistic stance when working with a client who self-harms will usually involve drawing on other theoretical orientations. For example, CBT techniques such as challenging distorted thinking, breathing techniques, and visualisations can be helpful. The visualisation can incorporate images of a safe, peaceful place when the client feels the urge to self-harm. This technique can be facilitated in therapy and practised in between sessions. Another approach is narrative therapy, and the client could be supported to tell their own story around their self-harm (Hoffman & Kress, 2008).

The client is encouraged to contribute to therapy goals, helping balance the power in the therapeutic relationship. The onus for progression is then shared between the client and the therapist, replacing the therapist's personal understanding and expectation of their view of progression. For example, a therapist may view cessation as the only indication of progression, having an agenda for change, whilst the client may view engaging in harm-minimisation techniques as a step towards healing. Other examples of goals the client may want to set and, if achieved, may view this as progression include them stating:

- "I want to understand why I self-harm"?
- "I want to talk about my feelings around my self-harm."
- "I want to stop but can only do this in stages."

It is crucial that the client feels respected and understood in how they perceive their self-harm and what they want to achieve in therapy. By feeling they are not being judged will avoid exacerbating their pain and, most likely, the severity of their self-harm. If the client can go at their own pace, they will hopefully stop self-harming at some point.

Some clients who self-harm may experience shame, finding it difficult to talk about their behaviour or may avoid eye contact with the therapist. Pluralistic sand-tray therapy can be a helpful way for the client to talk about their thoughts and feelings regarding their self-harming experience. They will focus on the sand display and project onto the objects, helping them work through their experience.

References

Abbing, A., Baars, E. W., De Sonneville, Ponstein, A. S. & Swaab, H. .(2019). The effectiveness of art therapy for anxiety in adult women: A randomized controlled trial. *Frontiers in Psychology: Psychology for Clinical Settings.* https://doi.org/10.3389/fpsyg.2019.01203 Retrieved February 2021.

Aldrich, C. K. (1974). Some dynamics of anticipatory grief. In B. Schoenberg, A. C. Carr, D. Peretz, & A. H. Kutscher (Eds.), *Anticipatory grief.* New York: Columbia University Press.

Allen, J. P., & Land, D. (1999). Attachment in adolescence. In J. Cassidy & P. R. Shaver (Eds.), *Handbook of attachment: Theory, research, and clinical applications* (pp. 319–335). New York: Guilford Press.

Aloi, J. A. (2009). Nursing the disenfranchised: Women who have relinquished an infant for adoption. *Journal of Psychiatric and Mental Health Nursing, 16*(1), 27–31.

Andover, M. S., Pepper, C. M., Ryabchenko, K. A., Orrico, E. G., & Gibb, B. E. (2005). Self-mutilation and symptoms of depression, anxiety and borderline personality order. *Suicide and Life-Threatening Behaviour, 35,* 581–591.

Barker, M. J. (2016). Helping clients improve their interpersonal relationships. In M. Cooper & W. Dryden (Eds.), *The handbook of pluralistic counselling and psychotherapy* (Chapter 16, pp. 198–210). London: Sage.

Beck, A. T. (1967). *Depression: Causes and treatment.* Philadelphia, PA: University of Pennsylvania Press.

Birditt, K. S., Miller, L. M., Fingerman, K. L., & Lefkowitz, E. S. (2009). Tensions in the parent and adult child relationship: Links to solidarity and ambivalence. *Psychology and Aging, 24*(2), 287–295.

Boisvert, M. M., Wright, J., Tremblay, N., & McDuff, P. (2011). Couples' reports of relationship problems in a naturalistic therapy setting. *The Family Journal: Counseling and Therapy for Couples and Families, 19*(4), 362–368.

Boss, P. (2000). *Ambiguous loss: Learning to live with unresolved grief.* Cambridge, MA: Harvard University Press.

Boss, P. (2010, April). The trauma and complicated grief of ambiguous loss. *Pastoral Psychology, 59*(2), 137–145.

Bradshaw, J. (2005). *Healing the shame that binds you* (2nd ed.). Deerfield Beach, FL. Health Communications.

Bridge, J. A., Goldstein, T. R., & Brent, D. A. (2006). Adolescent suicide and suicidal behaviour. *Journal of Child Psychology and Psychiatry, 47,* 372–394.

Brown, B. (2006). Shame resilience theory: A grounded theory study on women and shame. *Families in Society: The Journal of Contemporary Social Service, 87*(1), 43–52.

Bucx F., & van Wel, F. (2008). Parental bond and life course transitions from adolescence to young adulthood. *Family Therapy*, *35*, 109–126.

Childers, L. B. (Spring, 2010). Parental bonding in father-son relationships. Senior Honors Theses. 115. Liberty University. https://digitalcommons.liberty.edu/honors/115

Collins English Dictionary. HarperCollins Publishers. www.collinsdictionary.com/dictionary/english/anticipatory-loss Retrieved 15th February 2021.

Cooper, M., & Dryden, W. (2016). *Handbook of pluralistic counselling and psychotherapy*. In M. Cooper & W. Dryden (Eds.). London: Sage.

Cooper, M., & McLeod, J. (2011). *Pluralistic counselling and psychotherapy*. London: Sage.

Davidson, D. (2017). Art embodied: Tattoos as memorials. *Bereavement Care*, *36*(1), 33–40. DOI: 10.1080/02682621.2017.1305055

Dearing, R., Stuewig, J., & Tangney, J. (2005). On the importance of distinguishing shame from guilt: Relations to problematic alcohol and drug use. Addictive Behaviors, *30*, 1392–1404.

de Shazer, S., Berg, K., Lipchik, E., Nunnally, E., Molnar, A., Gingerich, W., & Weiner-Davis, M. (1986). Brief therapy: Focused solution development. *Family Process*, *25*(2), 207–222.

Doka, K. (1989). *Disenfranchised grief, recognising hidden sorrow*. Lexington, MA: Lexington Books.

Doss, B. D., Simpson, L. E., & Christensen, A. (2004). Why do couples seek marital therapy? *Professional Psychology: Research and Practice*, *35*, 608–614.

Dryden, W. (2016). Helping clients address problematic anxiety. In M. Cooper & W. Dryden (Eds.), *The handbook of pluralistic counselling and psychotherapy* (Chapter 15, pp. 173–183). London: Sage.

Farrell, A., & Geist-Martin, P. (2005). Communicating social health: Perceptions of wellness at work. *Management Communication Quarterly*, *18*, 543–592.

Fergusson, D. M., Woodward, L. J., & Horwood, L. J. (2000). Risk factors and life processes associated with the onset of suicidal behavior during adolescence and early adulthood. *Psychological Medicine*, *30*(1), 23–39.

Fingerman, K. L. (2001). *Aging mothers and their adult daughters: A study in mixed emotions*. New York: Springer Publishing Company.

Fleet, D., & Mintz, R. (2012). Counsellors' perceptions of client progression when working with clients who intentionally self-harm and the impact such work has on the therapist. *Counselling and psychotherapy research*, 1–9. http://doi.org/10.1080/14733145.2012.698421

Fleet, D. (2019). *Transformation hidden in the sand: Developing a theoretical framework using a sand-tray intervention with adult clients*. Doctoral thesis. Staffordshire University. Stoke-on-Trent. Available from Ethos STORE – Staffordshire Online Repository. https://eprints.staffs.ac.uk/id/eprint/5763

Fossum, M. A., & Mason, M. J. (1986). *Facing shame: Families in recovery*. London: W. W. Norton.

Frankl, V. (1962). *Man's search for meaning*. New York: Touchstone Books.

Gardner, F. (2001). *Self-harm: A psychotherapeutic approach*. London: Routledge, Taylor & Francis Group.

Geiss, S. K., & O'Leary, K. D. (1981). Therapist ratings of frequency and severity of marital problems: Implications for research. *Journal of Marital and Family Therapy*, *7*, 515–520.

Gendlin, E. T. (1984). *The client's client: The edge of awareness*. In R. L. Levant & J. M. Shlien (Eds.), *Client-centered therapy and the person-centered approach: New directions in theory, research and practice*. New York: Praeger.

Gillies, J., & Neimeyer, R. A. (2006). Loss, grief, and the search for significance: Toward a model of meaning reconstruction in bereavement. *Journal of Constructivist Psychology, 19*, 31–65.

Gilligan, J. (1997). *Violence: Reflections on a national epidemic*. New York: Vintage Books.

Gliatto, M. F., & Rai, A. K. (1999, March). Evaluation and treatment of patients with suicidal ideation. *American Family Physician, 59*(6), 1500–1506.

Graham, M. C. (2014). *Facts of life: Ten issues of contentment*. Parker, Colorado. Outskirts Press.

Greenberger, D., & Padesky, C. A. (1995). *Mind over mood: Change how you feel by changing the way you think*. New York: Guildford Press.

Greif, G. (2016, September 27). FAMILY DYNAMICS. 5 Key issues in difficult adult sibling relationships: This is what C should focus on when working with sibling issues. *Psychology Today*. www.psychologytoday.com/gb/blog/buddy-system/201609/5-key-issues-in-difficult-adult-sibling-relationships Retrieved 23 February 2021.

Hammerton, G., Mahedy, L., Mars, B., Harold, G. T., Thapar, A., Zammit, S., & Collishaw, S. (2015). Association between maternal depression symptoms across the first eleven years of their child's life and subsequent offspring ideation. PLOS ONE 10(8): e 0136367 doi.org/10.1371/journal.pone.0136367

Hammerton, G., Zammit, S., Mahedy, L., Pearson, R. M., Sellers, R., Thapar, A., & Collishaw, S. (2015). Pathways to suicide-related behavior in offspring of mothers with depression: The role of offspring psychopathology. *Journal of American Academy of Child & Adolescent Psychiatry, 54*(5), 385–393.

Hasseldine, R. (2020). Uncovering the root cause of mother-daughter conflict. American Counseling Association. file:///Users/doreenfleet/Desktop/Emotion%20&%20Relationships/Uncovering%20the%20root%20cause%20of%20mother-daughter%20conflict%20-%20Counseling%20Today.htm Retrieved 22 February 2021.

Hoffman, R., & Kress, V. (2008). Narrative therapy and non-suicidal-self-injurious behavior: Externalizing the problem and internalizing personal agency. *The Journal of Humanistic Education and Development, 47*(2). doi.org/10.1002/j.2161-1939.2008.tb00055.x

Jefferson, T. [1743–1826] https://founders.archives.gov Retrieved 12 April 2021.

Kubler-Ross, E. (1969). *On death and dying*. New York: Scribner.

Laye-Gindhu, A., & Schonert-Reichl, K. A. (2005). Nonsuicidal self-harm among community adolescents: Understanding the "whats" and "whys" of self-harm. *Journal of Youth and Adolescence, 34*(5), 447–457.

Levenson, R. W., Carstensen, L. L., & Gottman, J. M. (1993). Long-term marriage: Age, gender, and satisfaction. *Psychology and Aging, 8*, 301–313.

Lewis, H. B. (1971). Shame and guilt in neurosis. New York: International University Press.

Lindemann E. (1944). Symptomatology and management of acute grief. *American Journal of Psychiatry, 101*, 141–148.

McLeod, J. (2016). Helping clients address depression. In M. Cooper & W. Dryden (Eds.), *The handbook of pluralistic counselling and psychotherapy* (Chapter 14, pp. 173–183). London: Sage.

Michel, K., & Valach, L. (2011). The narrative interview with the suicidal patient. In K. Michel & D. A. Jobes (Eds.), Building a therapeutic alliance with the suicidal patient (pp. 63–80). *American Psychological Association*. https://doi.org/10.1037/12303-004

National Cancer Institute. Types of grief reactions. National Cancer Institute. http://ncinagpur.in/www.cancer.gov/about-cancer/advanced-cancer/caregivers/planning/bereavement-hp-pdq#section/all Retrieved 15 February 2021.

Neimeyer, R. A. (2016). Helping clients find meaning in grief and loss. In M. Cooper & W. Dryden (Eds.), *The handbook of pluralistic counselling and psychotherapy* (Chapter 17, pp. 211–222) London: Sage.

Parkes, C. M. (1996). *Bereavement* (2nd ed.). London & New York: Routledge.

Paulus, F. M., Müller-Pinzler, L., Jansen, A., Gazzola, V., & Krach, S. (2014). Mentalizing and the role of the posterior superior temporal sulcus in sharing others' embarrassment. *Cerebral Cortex*, *25*(8), 2065–2075.

Pembroke, L. (Ed.) (1996). Self-harm: Perspectives from personal experience. London Survivors Speak Out.

Pine, V. R. (1974). Dying, death and social behaviour. In B. Schoenberg, A. C. Carr, D. Peretz, & A. H. Kutscher (Eds.), *Anticipatory grief*. New York: Columbia University Press.

Rayner, C., & Cooper, C. L. (2006). Workplace bullying. In E. Kelloway, J. Barling, & J. Hurrell Jr. (Eds.), *Handbook of workplace violence* (pp. 47–90). Thousand Oaks, CA: Sage.

Reeves, A. (2010). Counselling suicidal clients (Therapy in practice). London: Sage Publications Ltd.

Reeves, A. (2015). Working with risk in counselling and psychotherapy. London: Sage Publications Ltd.

Reeves, A. (2017). In a search for meaning: challenging the accepted know-how of working with suicide risk. British Journal of Guidance & Counselling, *45*(5), 606–609.

Ritchie, H., & Roser, M. (2018). Mental health. Published online at OurWorldInData.org. Retrieved from https://ourworldindata.org/mental-health [online resource] Retrieved February 2021.

Royal College of Psychiatrists. (2020). Bereavement. Royal College of Psychiatrists: Public Engagement Editorial Board. www.rcpsych.ac.uk/mental-health/problems-disorders/bereavement Retrieved. 10 April 2021.

Rynearson, E. K., & Salloum, A. (2011). Restorative retelling: Revisiting the narrative of violent death. In R. A. Neimeyer, D. Harris, H. Winokuer, & G. Thornton (Eds.), *Grief and bereavement in contemporary society: Bridging research and practice* (pp. 177–188). New York: Routledge.

Sanderson, C. (2006). Counselling Adult Survivors of Child Sexual Abuse. London and Philadelphia: Jessica Kingsley Publishers.

Shaw, C., & Shaw, T. (2007). Chapter one: A dialogue of hope and survival. In H. Spandler & S. Warner (Eds.), *Beyond fear and control: Working with young people who self-harm*. Ross-on-Wye: PCCS Books.

Spandler, H., & Warner, S. (2007). Beyond fear and control: Working with young people who self-harm. Ross-on-Wye: PCCS Books.

Stavrianopoulos, K., & Faller, G., & Furrow, J. L. (2015). Emotionally focused family therapy: Facilitating change within a family system. *Journal of Couples & Relationship Therapy*, *13*, 25–43.

Swann-Thomas, B., Fleming, S., & Buckley, E. (2021). Etched in the skin: Grief on a living canvas memorial tattoos as expressions of grief. *Mortality*. DOI: 10.1080/13576275.2020.1865893

Tangney, J. P., & Dearing, R. (2002). *Shame and guilt.* New York: Guilford Press.

Taylor, E. R. (2009). Sandtray and solution-focused therapy. *International Journal of Play Therapy*, *18*(1), 56–68.

Trepper, T. S., McCollum, E. E., De Jong, P., Korman, H., Gingerich, W., & Franklin, C. (2010). Solution focused therapy treatment manual for working with individuals. Hammond, IN: Research Committee of the Solution Focused Brief Therapy Association. p. 1. www.andrews.edu/sed/gpc/faculty-research/coffen-research/trepper_2010_solution.pdf Retrieved 13 April 2021.

Turp, M. (1999). Encountering self-harm in psychotherapy and counselling practice. *British Journal of Psychotherapy*, *15*(3), 306–321.

Walsh, B. W. (2008). *Treating self-injury: A practical guide.* London: Guilford Press.

World Health Organization. (2017). *Depression and other common mental disorders: Global health estimates.* Geneva: World Health Organization. https://apps.who.int/iris/bitstream/handle/10665/254610/WHO-MSD-MER-2017.2-eng.pdf?sequence=1&isAllowed=y Retrieved 21 February 2021.

Yildirim, A., & Yildirim, D. (2007). Mobbing in the workplace by peers and managers: Mobbing experienced by nurses working in healthcare facilities in Turkey and its effect on nurses. *Journal of Clinical Nursing*, *16*(8), 1444–1453.

Chapter 10

Pluralistic sand-tray therapy with different client groups

Civilisations should be measured by the degree of diversity attained and the degree of unity maintained

(W. H. Auden https://best-quotations.com)

Every group in a society deserves the right to have access to therapy that is both supportive and non-judgemental. This chapter will discuss the diversity in client groups based on age, ethnicity, and gender presenting for therapy and explore how each group may benefit from pluralistic sand-tray therapy.

Age groups

The issue of mental health is an increasing global concern across all age groups. The World Health Organization (Ritchie & Roser, 2018) published data on mental health and estimated that "970 million people across the world had a mental or substance use disorder in 2017" (https://ourworldind ata.org/mental-health Retrieved 27 February 2021). Furthermore, in 2017, one in eight (12.8%) of 5- to 19-year-olds in the UK had at least one mental disorder (NHS Digital, 2018 https://digital.nhs.uk/ Retrieved 1/2/2021).

However, a review by The Lancet (Lola et al., 2021) indicated far higher figures of global psychological distress due to the COVID-19 pandemic. Lola et al. (2021) stated how current literature "shows high rates of psychological distress and early warning signs of an increase in mental health disorders" (p. 535).

People from every age category may seek or be guided to therapy for various reasons and problems they may be experiencing. Therefore, the question could be asked, "which age group benefits most from therapy"? Clarkin and Levy (2004), in line with Barber and Muenz's (1996) research, argued that age is not significant concerning therapeutic outcomes as all ages gain from having therapy. However, some research suggests some difference between the various age groups accessing therapy; Heisler et al. (1982) suggested that the dropout rate is higher for younger adults than older clients.

DOI: 10.4324/9781003158707-10

Agosti et al. (1996) supported this claim, arguing how younger clients with substance abuse disorders have poor retention and therapy outcomes. Furthermore, Sue and Lam (2002) suggested that older depressed clients benefited less from psychotherapy and Leaf et al. (1985) argued how older people are more reluctant to seek help than younger people.

The pluralistic sand-tray approach adopts a collaborative, flexible, and creative way of working with clients of all ages. Castonguay and Beutler (2005) appear to support this stance and stated, "The therapist is likely to increase" their "effectiveness if" they "demonstrate attitudes of open-mindedness, flexibility and creativity" (www.oxfordclinicalpsych.com Retrieved 11 March 2021). Besides, the pluralistic approach based on humanistic principles assumes that "the client is an active agent of change ..." (Cooper & McLeod, 2011, p. 18), contributing to building a collaborative and empathic relationship. Castonguay and Beutler (2005) argued how the therapist offering empathy is congruent and has an attitude that is warm and caring also contributes to the process of change for the client.

Adolescents

Adolescence is a critical stage in human development when emotional pressures and increased biological changes impact the individual (Shen & Armstrong, 2008). This transition, characterised by rapid changes, exists between childhood and maturity, which can be one of inner turmoil and social pressure. Schwarz (2009) suggested how adolescent clients can present for therapy due to experiencing a wide range of issues, including relationship problems, bullying, depression, generalised anxiety, suicidal ideation, and self-harm (Schwarz, 2009).

Ritchie and Roser (2018) suggested that mental health disorders become more evident during the stage of adolescence. Substance misuse factors are an additional risk to emotional pressures and biological changes (Ritchie & Roser, 2018) regarding adolescents' mental health. Bolton and Scherer (2003) argued how the prevalence and impact of mental health issues among adolescents are astonishing and stated, "Depression and depressive syndromes are common among adolescents" (Bolton & Scherer, 2003, p. 215) having severe repercussions, including "impaired social, academic, and occupational functioning" (Bolton & Scherer, 2003, p. 215).

Despite the apparent need to provide therapy for adolescents, Bolton and Scherer (2003) suggested that this client group is resistant to seeking therapy due to their developmental immaturity, the perceived stigma of going to therapy, and feeling coerced by adults into having therapy. Gallo-Lopez and Schaefer (2005) discussed how a therapist would need to consider creative approaches in counselling to meet the needs of adolescents. Bolton and Scherer (2003) argued that "establishing a strong therapeutic alliance with adolescents require that therapists express empathy and genuineness, utilise developmentally appropriate interventions, address the stigma, and increase choice in therapy" (p. 215).

Furthermore, the therapist must be genuine because adolescents, "particularly those in therapy, detest insincerity and pretence and often require a more directive approach" (Rubenstein, 1996). Candour is essential when helping the adolescent client engage, just as telling the truth is essential to building trust and establish a good therapeutic relationship (Sasson Edgette, 2001).

Adopting a directive and creative approach has been used in therapy when working with adolescents who have been sexually abused, depressed, or recovering from addiction (Veach & Gladding, 2007). Martinez and Lasser (2013) also argued that working creatively with adolescents is particularly useful when more traditional therapeutic approaches do not fit. However, it is essential that the therapist accepts the client's symbolism and avoids imposing their meaning onto any creative output (Allan, 1988).

Edgar-Bailey and Kress (2010) used a creative intervention with adolescents who had experienced a traumatic bereavement, which aided the therapeutic process. They explored the use of various creative interventions, including the adolescents finding objects that gave comfort (Edgar-Bailey & Kress, 2010). The objects kept as keepsakes helped the adolescents preserve the loved one's memory. Creative strategies such as working with pictures and objects help "decrease traumatic grief and facilitate the normal grieving process" (Edgar-Bailey & Kress, 2010, p. 172).

Sand tray is an expressive technique that invites adolescents to explore the uncertain world between childhood and adulthood, and Swank and Lenes (2013) viewed this approach to therapy as effective. Furthermore, Kestly (2005) suggested how sand tray could help adolescents explore identity development creatively, providing an appropriate balance between play therapy and traditional talking therapy. Such development issues include physical maturation, peer group relationships, and emotional development (Kail & Cavanaugh, 2016). Roaten (2011) argued how traditional talking therapy, usually based on adult rules, is likely to be ineffective with adolescents. However, with sand-tray therapy, a collaborative relationship helps the client take ownership of the therapeutic process (Roaten, 2011).

Pluralistic sand-tray therapy can be beneficial when working with adolescents in therapy. The pluralistic emphasis based on collaboration, setting goals, and working together focuses on establishing a two-way process, promoting a shared therapeutic relationship. In my experience as a therapist, many adolescents do not respond well to the non-directive and unstructured approach. Using structured sand-tray therapy can help the client become engaged as it gives a focus. As they engage in this creative therapy, it gives a sense of control, especially regarding eye contact. The client has the power to focus on the sand display or turn to look at the therapist sitting by the side of them. This way of working establishes a collaborative relationship between the therapist and the client, facilitating autonomy and freedom of expression for adolescents in the therapy.

Most of my adolescent clients have responded well to a structured sand-tray approach, especially in the early sessions. Once the client becomes familiar with the process and trust has been established, they often begin to take more control by stating how they know what they want to work on, using the sand tray at the beginning of a session. I find that when working with an adolescent, they usually want to hear the therapist express confidence about working with sand tray; at the beginning of the first session, it may help to comment:

> So when trying to talk about our feelings or about some difficult things we've experienced, it can sometimes help to work creatively.
>
> I have found that working with the sand tray and using the objects as symbols can be helpful, and I will help you talk about what you need to. There is no right way or wrong way to do this, only your way, so just do what feels right for you. You can also stop at any time if it is not working for you, and you can be honest with me because my aim is to help you. Have you got any questions you would like to ask me just now?

When suggesting a structured session, the examples in Chapter 6, such as "Eight emotions," "My givers and takers," and "Speaking the unspoken/unfinished business," can be useful depending on the client. However, a structured session may simply suggest that they create a sand display of how they perceive their problem, with the therapist helping them unpack that.

Young adults

The age span of younger adult clients is referred to as those aged between 18 and 39 years. A client from this age group spanning over 20 years can present with a myriad of problems and issues. Some examples include problems at work, relationship problems, bereavement, anxiety, depression, abuse, bullying, intentional self-harm, and suicide ideation. Due to this group's age span, there is likely to be a wide variation between clients; therefore, the therapist needs to avoid making assumptions and generalisations. For example, the client may be in a relationship and married, in a relationship and not married, or single; may work, may be unemployed, may be a full-time student, or a full-time carer for their children and family members; may be happy in their intimate relationship or may be in an abusive relationship. They may feel confident or not and have had a happy childhood or an abusive and neglected one. There are so many variables that it makes generalisations between these clients difficult.

The pluralistic approach is applicable here as the initial appointment will involve focusing on the issue to work on and indicate the client's goals and expectations and how best to work in therapy. The collaborative discussion between client and therapist will indicate if the client is happy to engage in pluralistic sand-tray therapy or not.

Clients in the mid-years

One definition of *midlife* is "the period of life between about 40–60" (Collins dictionary www.collinsdictionary.com/ Retrieved 10 March 2021). However, Jaques (1965) is noted to have identified the concept of *midlife crisis* and described this as "crises, which occur around the age of 35, which I shall term the mid-life crisis" (p. 502). Jaques (1965) suggested that this transition lasts for some years depending on the individual and, due to change in their biology, they are likely to experience misgivings, a loss of zest, and agonising inquiries. For example, the individual might become intensely aware of their limitations, diminishing options, and mortality. Lachman (2004) suggested that the stressors commonly associated with midlife include changes relating to menopause and "empty nest syndrome" when older children move out of the family home; although not significantly linked to midlife over other age brackets, it can be a time of stress and crisis.

However, over 50 years later, after Jaques's notion of the midlife crisis first emerged, life expectancy today is increasing, and what was considered middle-aged in the past no longer fits due to people living longer as a result of improved medicine and lifestyle changes. Thus, many people of 35 years and above have a younger and more active outlook, and the general expectations previously linked to midlife are inappropriate for this age bracket. For example, it is common for a person over 50 years to have a second career or engage in further education.

With this shift in age concept related to midlife, therapists must avoid making assumptions about such clients who come to therapy. For example, assuming the client is retired or moving towards retirement can be a barrier to forming a supportive relationship if they have a second career or are retraining and ambitious.

Murphy (2014) suggested that women in midlife who come for therapy might present with career issues, changes to their intimate relationships, problems in parenting adult children, and being in the role of caregivers to their parents. Other common problems include house moves, divorce, new family arrangements, and bereavement.

Some theorists now define an individual's age using two concepts of "chronological age" and "biological age." For example, Gian et al. (2019) defined an individual's "biological age as the individual physiological performance status that imperfectly correlates with chronological age. Chronological age equals the years a person has lived, and biological age is how old he or she seems, performs and/or feels" (p. 3).

Any judgement made by a therapist based on a client's chronological age could be perceived as ageism, resulting in them feeling disempowered and misunderstood, which is not a good grounding to establish an empathic therapeutic relationship.

The World Health Organization identified how a balance between work and leisure is essential for an adult's well-being and suggested how people from poor socio-economic backgrounds or the unemployed are at higher risk of developing a mental health disorder (Ritchie & Roser, 2018). In addition, supportive community structures can reduce the risk of developing a mental health disorder. However, individuals who do not have this social support can experience social exclusion and live in neighbourhoods where there is a high level of violence and crime, resulting in a higher risk of developing mental health disorders (Ritchie & Roser, 2018).

Steffen (2007) argued how "awareness of lifespan development is essential for Counselling Psychologists in order to contextualize their client's experiences and use this understanding as a resource for therapeutic work" (p. 21). It is also essential for therapists to be aware of death, death anxiety, and how it can impact a client's life, with death and mortality having a particular significance in midlife (Steffen, 2007).

However, Sugarman (2003) suggested how death awareness could add to an individual's lifespan awareness, assisting them to experience a different way of looking at an experience and adopting a different perspective.

For example, a client who had an intense fear of death at the beginning of therapy may move to a state of acceptance that every person will eventually die, so adopting a mindful attitude and living in the moment may bring new meaning and enjoyment into their life. Kübler-Ross (1975) embraced a positive view of death and stated how death was "the key to the door of life" (p. 164).

Pluralistic sand-tray therapy can be a valuable approach for midlife clients, with the tasks and methods adopted agreed in the initial assessment between client and therapist. Some clients in this age group will want to work in a non-structured way with them setting the agenda for each session, whilst others will want more direction. Purposeful dialogue in the assessment phase and the initial sand-tray session will establish a client's needs regarding whether they require direction or not to begin the process.

Older age group

The World Health Organization identified the older age group as having the highest risk of poor mental health, resulting from changes in life conditions, higher social exclusion, and loneliness (Ritchie & Roser, 2018). Furthermore, although bereavement is not restricted to older people, this experience is more common as people age. Ritchie and Roser (2018) discuss how, for this group, depression linked to bereavement is common. Other factors contributing to the risk of depression in older people include a decline in physical health and a decline in the individual's mobility and freedom (Ritchie & Roser, 2018). For example, an individual experiencing a stroke can result in dramatic implications, such as a decline in functional ability and upheaval in their personal relationships, resulting in depression (Raue et al., 2017).

Such dramatic changes to an older person's life can have an adverse effect, risking an increase in developing depression (Raue et al., 2017). These considerable losses can impact their self-concept, and they may perceive the changes as almost too much to bear. Sirey et al. (2008) argued that suicide rates are higher in older groups than younger groups.

Wuthrich and Frei (2015) suggested that various psychotherapies are helpful when working with depression in the older age group, and tailoring therapy to meet the individual's needs is required.

The literature suggests that some issues are common with older people coming to therapy. However, the therapist will need to keep in mind that each older person is a unique individual and may not conform to any generalised view of older people. A pluralistic stance takes this into account by tailoring the therapy to meet the client's needs and goals for therapy, such as incorporating Cognitive Behavioural Therapy (CBT) strategies to suit the client.

Some older people will be open to working creatively, whilst others will not.

Siampani (2013) described how she uses sand tray with older adults who have dementia. In her gestalt approach, Siampani stated, "I can only offer them the joy of creativity provided by the 'here and now', even when the human brain has lost some of its capacities" (p. 35). She argued how older clients in the initial or advanced stages of dementia could benefit from sand-tray therapy.

However, consideration needs to be given to a person over 60 who may be nearing the end of their working life, brought up a family, and may not be as flexible in their views when exploring their issues. It might be that they just want to tell their story and have somebody to listen, without giving an opinion. Alternatively, it might be that they feel the best way to solving their issue is to problem-solve.

Some older clients may think it quite infantile to work creatively when exploring their experience; therefore, it is crucial in the initial appointment to offer other ways of working that suit that specific client. It can also help to offer a more mature perspective on using the sand tray by using adult language and giving examples of how it has been effective for other older clients. Furthermore, the pluralistic approach can draw on other methods when therapists and clients establish the therapy tasks.

In my practice, I introduce the notion of sand-tray therapy to an older client by explaining how the objects act as physical metaphors to represent our experience, just as we use verbal metaphors in our speech. I will also offer an example of a verbal metaphor to clarify its meaning (Chapter 7). In my experience, this cognitive description communicates how sand-tray therapy is a legitimate way of working for adults in therapy, and most adult clients will then consider this option.

In the case study (Fleet, 2019), when Anne was first invited to use the sand-tray, she responded by laughing in embarrassment. However, once I informed her how using the objects as physical metaphors had helped other adults talk about some difficult issues, she became interested and decided she would like to see if this way of working could help her. The first therapy session was a profound experience for Anne, and at the end of therapy, she was surprised how well it had worked beyond her expectations.

Gender

The Human Rights Campaign defines the concept of gender as "One's inner-most concept of self as male, female, a blend of both or neither – how individuals perceive themselves and what they call themselves. One's gender identity can be the same or different from their sex assigned at birth" (www.hrc.org/ Retrieved 17 March 2021). The LGBT Foundation (2017) defined gender as "your internal sense of self, who you feel you are whether that's male, female or perhaps you don't feel strongly to any particular label about gender" (http:// lgbt.foundation/ Retrieved 17 March 2021).

Addis and Mahalik (2003) suggested how men seek help for their emotional and psychological distress far less than females do, and Collier (1982), in agreement, discussed how one in seven men compared to one in three women sought help from a mental health professional.

Similarly, Kessler et al. (1981) found that when men and women had similar emotional problems, women sought help significantly more than men did. Bowman (2008) described how males are less willing to self-disclose than women, which could impact men's reluctance to seek therapy.

Furthermore, Prager (1995) suggested how reluctance to self-disclose is a barrier to open dialogue, a core feature of therapy. Individuals who are members of the LGBTQ* community experience many destructive issues such as discrimination, bullying (Goodrich & Luke, 2015), genderism, and internalised homophobia (Farmer & Byrd, 2015), impacting whether they access counselling for their emotional and psychological distress.

Female clients

Gender roles are becoming increasingly androgynous (Gray et al., 2005, p. 351), yet gender socialisation still exists for both men and women, impacting the therapeutic process. Kaplan (1979) argued how women are socialised to be nurturing and emotional, and any achievement linked to affiliation with others. Mintz and O'Neil (1990) found that research suggested how "women are also hypothesised to be more open and affectively orientated in therapy than are men due to gender role socialization" (p. 382). Kaplan (1979) argued that women are likely to assume the subordinate role in the therapeutic relationship due to socialisation. Such power imbalance could negatively impact the female client, who may feel unable to question or challenge the therapist and may tend to please rather than get their needs met.

However, although gender role socialisation is still pervasive in contemporary society, the therapist will need to remain aware that female clients are not uniform in their characteristics. Some female clients, especially of a younger age, may not conform to the traditional gender stereotype. However, they still live in a society where others will have certain expectations of how females should behave and look in physical appearance, impacting their emotional and psychological state.

Some research has suggested how female clients had better outcomes in therapy that was supportive, was less challenging, and encouraged a trusting and collaborative relationship, rather than a confrontational one and discussed how women bring their gendered self into therapy (Stevens-Smith, 1995). Even so, therapists need to respect the differences between female clients when offering therapy. In addition, both male and female therapists need to be aware of a tendency toward gender bias based on traditional gender roles (Thorn & Page, 2004) and have a transparent attitude in clinical supervision to help foster a non-judgmental and empathic approach when working with female clients.

Norcross and Wampold (2011) argued how goal consensus, collaboration, and positive regard were effective elements of psychotherapy, and these aspects are compatible with pluralistic therapy. Ogrodniczuk et al. (2001) also suggested how female clients favoured a more directive approach with the counsellor advising how to work in therapy, and the therapist will need to consider this if a female client is seeking more direction.

Klagsbrun et al. (2005) investigated how female participants experienced working creatively in therapy. All the participants commented on how working creatively was restorative, uplifting, and energising and perceived improvements in their overall quality of life due to creative therapy.

In my practice, pluralistic sand-tray therapy has been successful with many female clients, the vast majority who readily accepted the invitation to work in this way. The research contribution from Ogrodniczuk et al. (2001) suggesting that female clients favour more direction can be addressed in pluralistic sand-tray therapy by adopting a structured sand-tray approach (Chapter 6). The therapist can offer an intervention depending on the current issue the client needs to explore. However, it is vital to keep in mind that some female clients will want to work in an unstructured way.

Male clients

Seidler et al. (2018) reported how research suggests that many men are reticent to seek therapy, and when they do, the drop out rate is high (Spendelow,

2015). Also, men who have had therapy, frequently perceive it as a negative experience, which risks them not seeking therapy for their mental health in the future (Syzdek et al., 2016).

Basow (1986) suggested how gender roles indicating a difference in the socialisation of men and women have become established in society. Men are often perceived as emotionally inhibited, independent and associate sexuality with self-esteem and manliness (Gilbert, 1987). Maracek and Johnson (1980) argued how evidence shows that men show less affect in therapy than women. Mintz and O'Neil (1990) advise how therapists will need to be aware of male clients who conform to traditional, nontraditional or of a particular ethnic background and adapt their approach to build an effective therapeutic relationship.

However, "many men have a sceptical attitude toward therapy, and we find this tendency to be even more pronounced among working-class men, asking for help or admitting weakness are inconsistent with masculinity" (Gray et al., 2005, p. 352). Brooks (1998) took a similar stance and argued how talking about feelings and confronting pain does not sit easily with traditional male traits. However, Seidler et al. (2018) were critical of the deficit-based view of why men have negative experiences and are reluctant to seek therapy. Instead, they emphasised clinicians who are biased against masculinity and suggested that it was necessary to ensure they have adequate training in gender socialisation. Seidler et al. (2019) recommended adapting the clinical environment, therapy content, and therapeutic relationship by making it more men-centred. This would involve adaptations such as clinical training in gender socialisation, breaking down treatment options and their constituents, establishing short-term goals for therapy, and facilitating a balanced, collaborative therapeutic relationship (Seidler et al., 2018). These adaptations are conducive to the pluralistic approach that emphasises collaboration, establishing goals and tasks of therapy, and includes the client in any decision.

Pluralistic sand-tray therapy can facilitate a male client to connect and express their feelings in a way that talking therapy alone does not. The symbolism and projection on to the objects in the sand and the mechanism of touch aids emotional expression.

This argument supported by research suggests how sand-tray therapy is associated with emotional expression (Bradway & McCoard, 1997; Homeyer & Sweeney, 2011; Turner, 2005).

LGBTQ* clients

The acronym "LGBTQ* stands for lesbian, gay, bisexual, transgender queer and questioning. These terms are used to describe a person's sexual orientation or gender identity" (https://gaycenter.org/ Retrieved 26 March 2021). Discrimination (Goodrich & Luke, 2015), genderism, and internalised homophobia could result in an LGBTQ individual being reluctant to seek therapy (Farmer & Byrd, 2015). Genderism is defined as "the cultural belief that gender is binary, or that there are, or should be only two genders, man and woman, and that the aspects of one's gender are inherently linked to the sex in which they were assigned at birth" (https://psychology.wikia.org Retrieved 26 March 2021).

Destructive attitudes might cause a person from the LGBTQ* community to question whether therapy could help them, asking themselves questions such as "can this therapist be non-judgemental with me"? or "will I be understood if the therapist does not have an awareness of who I am"? which may be a barrier to accessing therapy.

Boughey (2021) discussed how genderism is an issue and shared how some of his LGBTQ* clients have had negative experiences with previous therapists. One issue involved some clients having to justify why they think they are gay, leaving them feeling misunderstood and judged. Another issue involved the struggle to find a therapist who is part of the LGBTQ* community because the client perceived they would be understood and not judged by them.

Therapists who are not part of the LGBTQ* community and aim to offer therapy to clients will need multicultural competence. They will also need to be prepared to work transparently and reflexively in clinical supervision so that any sign of genderism or internalised discrimination can be challenged and processed. Such supervision is likely to increase the therapist's ability to support marginalised communities (Garza-Chaves et al., 2018).

Utilising creativity in therapy has been effective when working with various populations, including the LGBTQ* community (Gladding, 2010; Paone et al., 2015). Sand-tray therapy is an example of creative therapy exploring intra- and interpersonal issues (Isom et al., 2015).

A client who is from a marginalised group is likely to have experienced some form of discrimination, which can disempower the individual. Thus, the collaborative nature of pluralistic sand-tray therapy intends to respect the client's autonomy and values their knowledge and skills when deciding what their goals are and how they and their therapist will work together. This way of working for an LGBTQ* client, setting the agenda for each sand-tray session, is an affirming approach that can equalise the power balance between client and therapist.

Ethnicity and race

Ramsey (2014) stated, "In this time of increasing globalisation, it is not uncommon to practice counseling in a context with native speakers of multiple languages" (p. 541). Clarkin and Levy (2004) suggested that clients from varying ethnic backgrounds have mostly equally good therapeutic outcomes. Nevertheless, Beutler et al. (2006) argued that clients from African-American backgrounds have poor outcomes than clients from other ethnic groups. Zane et al. (2004) suggested how Asian American clients were less satisfied with therapy than white clients. However, Sue et al. (2009) found "disparities in the quality of services delivered to ethnic minority groups" (p. 525) and reported that research evidence suggests that cultural competency in therapy is valuable and needed. "Therapists must be able to communicate with clients in a manner that is culturally acceptable and appropriate" (Sue et al., 2009, p. 534).

Griner and Smith (2006) provided evidence for the value of cultural competency therapy with clients from ethnic backgrounds. A culturally competent therapist is more likely to overcome cultural barriers. The more they know about a client from a diverse ethnic background, including the discrimination they experience, the more at ease the client will be in therapy.

Based on case studies, Ramsey's (2014) research concluded a stage model using sand-tray therapy with Albanian clients from various educational and economic backgrounds. The first stage identified as the Building phase, which incorporated the client to explore their inner thoughts, feelings, self-identity, memories, and hesitations (p. 543), which were made visible by creating a display in the sand. The next stage, the Bonding stage, involved the client sharing their awareness of each object, encouraging subconscious projection. The Being stage occurred when both client and therapist "work with the inner world of the client in the here and now" (p. 543), involving acting out and interaction between the objects to help foster insight. The final session focused on facilitating the client to name their world, pictured in the sand tray, which had the effect of summarising the process for the client.

Ramsey (2014) suggests how sand-tray therapy enables the exploration of non-verbal and pre-verbal material. The therapist adopts the role of "visitor" to the client's inner world. The sand-tray image is the client's visual interpretation of their experience, which can aid their vocabulary and culture-based assumptions are shared (Ramsey, 2014). Ramsey stated, "It provides a cultural window for insight in assessment and diagnosis and a bridge for the use of therapy techniques within the cultural context "(p. 541). In my own practice, when counselling clients from diverse ethnic backgrounds, I found it essential to have a range of objects that represented different cultures, and human figures need to represent clients from various ethnic backgrounds.

A word of caution concerning using the term "BAME" (Black, Asian, and Minority Ethnic), referred to in various literature and many institutions and groups: therapists need to be aware that not all people from diverse ethnic backgrounds perceive this term as positive. The argument is that it can mislead people into thinking that everyone who is not white English comes under the term "BAME." Therefore, it is essential to understand each client's story and how they see the world, empathy being key, so that individual does not feel judged and misunderstood. In addition, therapists need to stay updated with current literature and societal changes to what is deemed acceptable regarding using terms related to ethnicity.

Shirley, who was part of the case study (Chapter 2 and Chapter 4), described herself as Black African, and it was vital for me as a therapist to acknowledge and respect her way of perceiving her ethnicity and religious views by bracketing my own beliefs and opinions. Empathising with Shirley's frame of reference helped her feel accepted, and she was able to share and explore her fear and deep intrapsychic experience that contributed to her anxiety.

By the end of therapy, she had spoken out loud, something she had not been able to say before and was managing her anxiety more effectively, which was reinforced by her feedback and improvement in her CORE-10 clinical scores.

References

Addis, M. E., & Mahalik, J. R. (2003). Men, masculinity and the contexts of help seeking. *American Psychologist*, *58*, 5–14.

Agosti, V., & Nunes, E., & Ocepeck-Welikson, K. (1996). Client factors related to early attrition from outclient cocaine research clinic. *American Journal of Drug and Alcohol Abuse*, *22*, 29–39.

Allan, J. (1988). *Inscapes of the world*. Dallas, TX: Spring Publications.

Auden, W. H. (1907–1973). https://best-quotations.com Retrieved 12 April 2021.

Barber, J. P., & Muenz, L. R. (1996). The role of avoidance and obsessiveness in matching patients to cognitive and interpersonal psychotherapy: Empirical findings from the Treatment of Depression Collaborative Research Program. *Journal of Consulting Clinical Psychology*, *64*(5), 951–958.

Basow, S. A. (1986). *Gender stereotypes: Traditional and alternatives*. Monterey, CA: Brooks/Cole.

Beutler, L., Blatt, S. J., Alimohamed, S., Levy, K. N., & Angtuaco. L. (2006). Participant factors in dysphoric disorders. In L. G. Castonguay & L. E. Beutler (Eds.), *Principles of therapeutic change that work* (pp. 111–117). New York: Oxford University Press..

Bolton Oetzel, K., & Scherer, D. G. (2003). Therapeutic engagement with adolescents in psychotherapy. *Psychotherapy: Theory, Research, Practice, Training*, *40*(3), 215–225.

Bowman, J. M. (2008). Gender role orientation and relational closeness: Self-disclosure behaviour in same-sex male friendships. *The Journal of Men's Studies*, *16*, (3), 316–330.

Boughey, J. (2021). *Dialogue on genderism between Dr D. Fleet and J. Boughey*. (www.banishthecrows.co.uk). Retrieved 27 March 2021.

Bradway, K., & McCoard, B. (1997). *Sandplay: Silent workshop of the psyche*. New York: Routledge.

Brooks, G. (1998). *A new psychotherapy for traditional men*. San Francisco, CA: Jossey-Bass.

Castonguay, L. G., & Beutler, L. E. (2005). *Principles of therapeutic change that work*. New York: Oxford University Press. Published online July 2015. www.oxfordclinicalpsych.com/ Retrieved 11 March 2021.

Clarkin, J. F., & Levy, K. N. (2004). The influence of client variables on psycho-therapy. In M. J. Lambert (Ed.), *Bergin and Garfield's handbook of psychotherapy and behavior change* (5th ed., pp. 194–226). Chicago, IL: John Wiley & Sons.

Collier, H. V. (1982). *Counseling women: A guide for therapists*. New York. Macmillan.

Collins dictionary www.collinsdictionary.com/ Retrieved 10 March 2021.

Cooper, M. & McLeod, J. (2011). *Pluralistic Counselling and Psychotherapy*. London: Sage

Edgar-Bailey, M., & Kress, V. (2010). Resolving child and adolescent traumatic grief: Creative techniques and interventions. *Journal of Creativity in Mental Health*, *5*(2), 158–176. https://doi.org/10.1080/15401383.2010.4850090

Farmer, L. B., & Byrd, R. (2015). Genderism in the LGBTQQIA community: An interpretative phenomenological analysis. *Journal of LGBT Issues in Counseling*, *9*(4), 288–310.

Fleet, D. (2019). *Transformation hidden in the sand: Developing a theoretical frame-work using a sand-tray intervention with adult clients*. Doctoral thesis. Staffordshire University. Stoke-on-Trent. Available from Ethos STORE – Staffordshire Online Repository. https://eprints.staffs.ac.uk/id/eprint/5763

Gallo-Lopez, L., & Schaefer, C. E. (Eds.). (2005). *Play therapy with adolescents*. Lanham, MD: Jason Aronson.

Garza-Chaves, Y., Timm, N., & Oeffinger, J. (2018). Sand-tray, superheroes, and the healing journeys. *Journal of Counselor Practice*, *9*(1), 24–38.

Gian, A. R, Aldo, C., Sacchi, N., Castagnetta., Puntoni, M., Amaro, A., Banelli, B., & Pfeffer, U. (2019). Biological age versus chronological age in the prevention of age associated diseases. *OBM Geriatrics*, *3*(2).

Gilbert, L. A. (1987). Female and male emotional dependency and its implications for the therapist–client relationships. *Professional Psychology: Theory, Research and Practice*, *18*(6), 555–556.

Gladding, S. T. (2010). *The creative arts in counseling*. American Counseling Association.

Goodrich, K. M., & Luke, M. (2015). Group counseling with LGBTQI persons. *American Counseling Association*.

Gray Deering, C., & Gannon, E. J. (2005). Gender and psychotherapy with traditional men. *American Journal of Psychotherapy*, *59*(4), 351–360.

Griner, D., & Smith T. B. (2006). Culturally adapted mental health intervention: A meta-analytic review. *Psychotherapy: Theory, Research, Practice & Training*, *43*(4), 531–548.

Heisler, R. W., Beck. N. C., Fraps, C. L., & McReynolds, W. T. (1982). Therapist ratings as predictiors of therapy attendance. *Journal of Clinical Psychology*, *38*, 754–758.

Homeyer, L. E., & Sweeney, D. S. (2011). *Sandtray therapy: A practical manual* (2nd ed.). London: Routledge.

Isom, E. E., Groves-Radomski, J., & McConaha, M. M. (2015). Sandtray therapy: A familial approach to healing through imagination. *Journal of Bisexuality*, *10*(4), 429–451.

Jaques, E. (1965). Death and the mid-life crisis. *International Journal of Psycho-Analysis*, *46*, 502–514.

Kail, R. V., & Cavanaugh, J. C. (2016). *Human development: A life-span view* (7th ed.). Boston, MA: Cengage Learning.

Kaplan, A. G. (1979). Toward an analysis of sex-role related issues in the therapeutic relationships. *Psychiatry*, *43*, 112–120.

Kessler, R. C., Brown, R. L., & Boman, C. L. (1981). Sex differences in psychiatric help seeking: Evidence from four large-scale surveys. *Journal of Health Social Behavior*, *22*, 49–64.

Kestly, T. (2005). Adolescent sand tray therapy. In L. Gallo-Lopez & C. E. Schaefer (Eds.), *Play therapy with adolescents* (pp. 18–29). Lanham, MD: Jason Aronson.

Klagsbrun, J., Rappaport, L., Marcow Speiser, V., Post., Byers, J., Stepakoff, S., & Karman, S. (2005). Focusing and expressive arts therapy as a complementary treatment for women with breast cancer. *Journal of Creativity in Mental Health, 1*(1), 107–137.

Kübler-Ross, E. (1975). *Death: The final stage of growth.* New York: Touchstone.

Lachman, M. E. (2004). Development in midlife. *Annual Review of Psychology, 55,* 305–331.

Leaf, P. J., Livingston, M. M., Tischler, G. L., Weissman, M. M., Holzer, C. E., & Myers, J. K. (1985). Contact with health professionals for the treatment of psychiatric and emotional problems. *Medical Care, 23,* 1322–1337.

The Lesbian, Gay, Bisexual Transgender Community Center. What is LBGTQ? https://gaycenter.org/ Retrieved 26 March 2021.

LGBT Foundation (2017). http://lgbt.foundation Retrieved 17 March 2021.

Lola, K., Kohrt, B. A., Hanlon, C. et al. (2021). COVID-19 mental health impact and responses in low-income and middle-income countries: Reimagining global mental health. *The Lancet, 8,* 535–550. www.thelancet.com/psychiatry. Retrieved 25 June 2021.

Maracek, J., & Johnson, M. (1980). Gender and the process of therapy. In A. M. Brodsky & R. Hare-Mustin (Eds.), *Women and psychotherapy: An assessment of research and practice* (pp. 67–93). New York. Guildford Press.

Martinez, A., & Lasser, J. (2013). Thinking outside the box while playing the game: A creative school-based approach to working with children and adolescents. *Journal of Creativity in Mental Health, 8,* 81–91.

Mintz, L. B., & O'Neil, J. (1990). Gender roles, sex, and the process of psychotherapy: Many questions and few answers. *Journal of Counseling & Development, 68,* 381–387.

Murphy, S. N. (2014). Midcourse corrections. *Counseling Today: American Counseling Association.* 24 September 2014.

Norcross, J. C., & Wampold, B. E. (2011). Evidence-based therapy relationships: Research conclusions and clinical practices. In J. C. Norcross (Ed.), *Psychotherapy relationships that work: Evidence-based responsiveness* (2nd ed., pp. 3423–3430). New York: Oxford University Press.

Ogrodniczuk, J. S., Piper, W. E., Joyce, A. S., & McCallum, M. (2001). Effect of patient gender on outcome in two forms of short-term individual psychotherapy. *The Journal of Psychotherapy Practice and Research, 10,* 69–78.

Paone, T. R., Malott, K. M., Gao, J., & Kinda, G. (2015). Using sandplay to address students' reactions to multicultural counselor training. *International Journal of Play Therapy, 24*(4), 190–204.

Prager, K. J. (1995). *The psychology of intimacy.* New York. Guildford Press.

Psychology Wiki. Genderism. https://psychology.wikia.org Retrieved 26 March 2021.

Ramsey, L. C. (2014). Windows and bridges of sand: Cross-cultural counseling using sand tray methods. *Procedia – Social and Behavioral Sciences, 159,* 541–545.

Raue, P. J., McGovern, A. R., Dimitris, N., Kiosses, D. N., & Sirey, J. A. (2017). Advances in psychotherapy for depressed older adults. *Current Psychiatry Repository, 19*(9), 57.

Ritchie, H., & Roser, M. (2018). Mental health. Published online at OurWorldInData.org. Retrieved from https://ourworldindata.org/mental-health [online resource] Retrieved 27 February 2021. NHS Digital, 2018 https://digital.nhs.uk/ Retrieved 1/2/2021.

Roaten, G. K. (2011). Innovative and brain-friendly strategies for building a therapeutic alliance with adolescents. *Journal of Creativity in Mental Health*, 6, 298–314.

Rubenstein, A. K. (1996). Interventions for a scattered generation: Treating adolescents in the nineties. *Psychotherapy: Theory, Research, Practice, Training*, 33, 353–360.

Sasson Edgette, J. (2001). *Candor, connection, and enterprise in adolescent therapy*. New York: W. W. Norton.

Schwarz, S. W. (2009, June). *Facts for policymakers: Adolescent mental health in the United States*. National Center for Children in Poverty. Retrieved from www.nccp.org/publications/pdf/text_878.pdf

Seidler, Z., Rice, S. M., Ogrodniczuk, J. Oliffe, J. L., Shaw, J., & Dhillon, H. M. (2019). Men, Masculinities, Depression: Implications for Mental Health Services From a Delphi Expert Consensus Study. *Professional Psychotherapy: Research and Practice*. Advance online publication. http://dx.doi.org/10.1037/pro0000220

Seidler, Z. E., Rice, S. M., Ogrodniczuk, J. S., Oliffe, J. L., & Dhillon, H. M. (2018). Engaging men in psychological treatment: A scoping review. *American Journal of Men's Health*, 12(6), 1882–1900.

Shen, Y. P., & Armstrong, S. A. (2008). Impact of group sandtray therapy on the self-esteem of young adolescent girls. *The Journal for Specialists in Group Work*, 33(2), 118–137.

Sirey, J. A., Bruce, M. L., Carpenter, M., Booker, D., Reid, M. C., Newell, K. A., et al. (2008). Depressive symptoms and suicidal ideation among older adults receiving home delivered meals. *International Journal of Geriatric Psychiatry*, 23(12), 1306–1311.

Spendelow, J. S. (2015). Cognitive–behavioral treatment of depression in men: Tailoring treatment and directions for future research. *American Journal of Men's Health*, 9(2), 94–102.

Steffen, E. (2007). Death and mid-life: Why an understanding of life-span development is essential for the practice of counselling psychology. *Counselling Psychology Review*, 22(3), 21–25.

Stevens-Smith, P. (1995). Gender issues in counsellor education: Current status and challenges. *Counselor Education and Supervision*, 34(4), 283–294. doi:10.1002/j.1556-6978.1995.tb00195.x

Sue, S., & Lam, A. G. (2002). Cultural and demographic diversity. In J. Norcross (Ed.), *Psychotherapy relationships that work: Therapists relational contributors to effective psychotherapy* (pp. 401–421). New York: Oxford University Press.

Sue, S., Zane, N., Nagayama Hall, G. C., & Berger, L. K. (2009). The case for cultural competency in psychotherapeutic interventions. *Annual Review of Psychology*, 60, 525–548.

Sugarman, L. (2003). The life course as a meta-model. In R. Woolfe, W. Dryden, & S. Strawbridge (Eds.), *Handbook of counselling psychology* (pp. 303–321). London: Sage.

Swank, J. M., & Lenes, E. A. (2013). An exploratory inquiry of sandtray group experiences with adolescent females in an alternative school. *The Journal for Specialists in Group Work*, 38(4), 330–348.

Syzdek, M. R., Green, J. D., Lindgren, B. R., & Addis, M. E. (2016). Pilot trial of gender-based motivational interviewing for increasing mental health service use in college men. *Psychotherapy*, *53*(1), 124–129.

Thorn, C., & Page, S. (2004). Conceptualizations of health: A test of the theory of male bias. *Guidance and Counselling*, *20*(1), 64–70.

Turner, B. A. (2005). *The handbook of sandplay therapy*. Cloverdale, CA: Temenos Press.

Veach, L. J., & Gladding, S. T. (2007). Using creative group techniques in high schools. *The Journal for Specialists in Group Work*, *32*(1), 71–81.

Wuthrich, V. M., & Frei, J. (2015). Barriers to treatment for older adults seeking psychological therapy. *Journal of International Psychogeriatrics*, *27*(7), 1227–1236.

Zane, N., Hall, G. C. N., Sue, S., Young, K., & Nunez, J. (2004). Research on psychotherapy with culturally diverse populations. In M. J. Lambert (Ed.), *Bergin and Garfield's handbook of psychotherapy and behavior change* (5th ed., pp. 767–804). Chicago, IL: John Wiley & Sons.

Chapter 11

Clinical supervision of pluralistic sand-tray therapy

> Most people believe vulnerability is weakness. But really, vulnerability is courage. We must ask ourselves…are we willing to show up and be seen?
>
> (Bene Brown. www.pinterest.at/)

Carson and Becker (2004) stated, "most counsellors/therapists feel stuck in the counselling process with at least some clients some of the time" (p. 111). Therefore, it is vital that the therapist is courageous, willing to expose their vulnerability in clinical supervision and share their thoughts around feeling deskilled at times. Then with the help of the supervisor, this issue can be openly explored and resolved.

Any anxiety experienced by the supervisee can be exacerbated when feeling pressure to account for a decision they intend to make concerning their practice. For example, a supervisee may communicate that they want to incorporate a new or different way of working with their clients and are asked by the supervisor to justify this change. The supervisor needs to manage this issue, avoiding adopting an authoritarian attitude that may communicate their personal preference, dismissing the view of the supervisee. Instead, supervisors need to establish a tolerant and supportive relationship by openly facilitating development in the supervisee's practice.

Even for experienced therapists, there will be times when they feel de-skilled in supervision and experience "stuckness" with a client. Therefore, it is vital that the supervisor's support is non-judgemental, enabling the supervisee to bring difficulties they are experiencing with their clients. Lombardo, Milne, and Procter (2009) suggested how intense discussion in supervision can result in the supervisee feeling de-skilled and stresses the need for space for emotional processing. "It is not anxiety itself that is destructive, but the denial, repression or rationalising of it" (Dryden and Thorne, 1991, p. 90) and an empathic, supportive relationship is more conducive to exploring anxiety in a non-defensive manner.

There are various opinions on what is clinical supervision in counselling and psychotherapy. Milne and Watkins (2014) definition is "the formal

DOI: 10.4324/9781003158707-11

provision, by approved supervisors, of a relationship-based education and training that is work-focused and which manages, supports, develops and evaluates the work of colleague/s" (p. 4). However, the different theoretical approaches will emphasise various aspects of clinical supervision depending on their underpinning philosophies.

Cognitive behaviour clinical supervision

Cognitive behavioural supervision (CBS) tends to be structured, including feedback and evaluation of audiotapes and videotapes, live demonstration role-play rehearsal, and agenda discussions (Milne et al., 2010), with evidence-based practice a significant aspect of cognitive behavioural therapy (CBT). Structured supervision, including assessing the supervisee's work, is deemed to impact supervisees positively (Milne et al., 2010). Gorden's (2012) framework involves a collaborative discussion to clarify the supervision question to set the "agenda in supervision, just as in therapy" (p. 72). This collaboration strengthens the working alliance (Bordin, 1983). Other aspects incorporate "active problem-solving methods, checking if the supervision question has been answered" (Gorden, 2012, p. 78), forming action plans and feedback. CBT supervision focuses on specific competencies, guiding therapist training and assessing a therapist's clinical practice (Bernard & Goodyear, 1998), regarding evidence-based practice as essential. Examples of standardised coding instruments used to measure competencies include the "Cognitive Therapy Adherence and Competence Scale" (Barber et al., 2003) and the "Assessment of Core CBT Skills" (Muse et al., 2017).

Thus, in CBT, evidence-based practice is an essential feature regarding therapy and clinical supervision.

Person-centred therapy supervision

There is a striking difference between the person-centred approach (PCT) approach to supervision and other approaches. The PCT approach accentuates the personhood of the supervisee and their development (Lambers, 2013). When discussing the process of supervision, Carl Rogers suggested that the primary goal of supervision was to facilitate the supervisee to grow in self-confidence and develop their understanding of the therapeutic process (Hackney et al.,1984).

Furthermore, in 1983 Patterson argued how supervision is not therapy but turns out to be therapeutic via the supervisory relationship exemplifying empathy, respect, and genuineness. Thus, Patterson (1983) classified his approach "under the personal-emotional orientation (along with Rogers, Arbuckle and Atucher), which involves the supervisor as counselor" (p. 21). However, Patterson was also concerned "with the personal skills orientation" (p. 21) of PCT supervision.

Rice (1980) suggested there were two elements to PCT supervision, incorporating a "theory of process" and a "theory of relationship." The "theory of process" refers to supervisees bringing themselves as the focus of supervision and developing their therapeutic ability (Lambers, 2013). The "theory of relationship" emphasises the importance of the relationship between supervisor and supervisee (Ramos-Sánchez et al., 2002) based on empathy, congruence and acceptance. Similarly, Callifronas and Brock (2017) viewed the aim of supervision as "to respect the supervisee's own internal power and focus upon their personal and professional development" (p. 9) and to develop their skills using their own resources, epitomising the PCT approach.

Tally and Jones (2019) described how the PCT "supervisor structures the supervision around the supervisee's experience of the client and of their sessions together to facilitate the process of professional development within the counselor" (p.22). In addition, Mearns (1997) identified questions for the supervisee to reflect on during PCT supervision, including "What do I feel in relation to this client?" and "are there any blocks to my empathy with this client?" (p. 88).

These questions facilitate reflexivity in the supervisee, guiding further exploration. However, although PCT supervision is focused on the supervisee's potential, the supervisor still has the role of gatekeeper, responsible for challenging any unethical practice by the supervisee (Tally & Jones, 2019). For example, Tally and Jones (2019) discussed how Villas-Boas Bowen (2002) suggested that therapists who are not aware of their personal needs and fears, some of which may be unconscious, can negatively impact the client's process. Thus, Rogers's goal of helping supervisees develop their self-awareness and understanding of the therapeutic process was essential.

Gestalt supervision using creative interventions

Casado-Kehoe and Ybañez (2011) discussed how using creative interventions in gestalt supervision could enhance communication and develop the supervisee's therapeutic competence. The rationale for this argument is that symbolic representations can help the supervisee explore their inner and outer reality (Lahad, 2000). The physical picture or object aids the supervisee to explore their phenomenological experience in the "here and now," helping to increase awareness. Houston (2013) stated, "my job as a gestalt counselor is to raise awareness" (p. 15).

Similar to PCT theory, Gestalt proposes that people have the power to change by developing self-awareness (Beisser, 1970). This process named the "paradoxical theory of change" (Beisser, 1970), is concerned with the whole person and the context in which they are now and in their life; "so gestalt is holistic" (Houston, 2013, p. 16). The rationale is that change occurs when the person fully accepts what is now. The therapist will help the client stay focused on the present by directing their effort to escape the present by talking about the past and future (Houston, 2013). The goal is to develop the individual's holistic experience in the present moment (Sommers-Flanagan & Sommers-Flanagan, 2012). The therapist will stay alert to the behaviour of the client and themselves concerning breathing, posture, tension, voice tone, movements and hesitations" (Houston, 2013, p. 33).

In line with PCT, Gestalt fosters a caring, accepting, and non-judgmental attitude towards clients (Casado-Kehoe and Ybañez, 2011). The individual is helped to lower their resistance and become fully present by engaging the body, senses, emotions, and intellect as trust develops in the therapeutic relationship. Establishing this type of supportive relationship also applies to that between supervisor and supervisee.

When using creative interventions in supervision, the supervisee asked to try something during supervision aids the development of awareness and focuses on their thoughts, feelings, and physical sensations concerning their work with their clients. This development in awareness occurs via phenomenological dialogue involving them communicating their "internal, intrapsychic happenings that occur to them from moment to moment" (Houston, 2013 p. 57). For example, when using a creative intervention to explore the supervisee's response to a picture or symbolic object representing some aspect of their work with a client, helpful questions asked by the supervisor aid this process. Examples might be, "What are you feeling as you say that?" and "Where in your body do you register that feeling?" (Houston, 2013, p. 60) help increase awareness of the supervisee that will positively impact their work as therapists.

Pluralistic clinical supervision

Similar to CBT supervision, pluralistic clinical supervision is structured and incorporates pluralistic principles, including goal and agenda-setting, collaboration, and discussion on feedback (McLeod, 2018). Creaner and Timulak (2016, p. 314) stated, "good supervisors are flexible in their approach (Borders, 2014) and ethical in their practice (Thomas, 2007)", adopt a research attitude, committed to inclusive practice and engage in outcomes for the supervisee and the client.

However, Ellis (1991) argued that it is not uncommon for difficulties to occur during clinical supervision and supervisees to feel harmed following supervision. Sweeney & Creaner (2014) suggested how a good supervisory relationship would encourage the supervisee to self-disclose. However, a supervisee who believes they will be criticised is unlikely to share their anxiety about their work with their clients being fearful that they will be perceived as not capable by the supervisor. Ladany (2004) suggested some causes of problematic supervision include confrontational criticism, blaming, and unclear agendas. Therefore, an empathic, collaborative relationship involving setting goals, establishing an agenda for each session, with the supervisor acknowledging the supervisee's strengths without blame, can avoid such difficulties occurring. The PCT approach of prizing the supervisee, offering empathy, and being congruent are also essential features of pluralistic supervision.

Cooper (2019) described how he tries to get a sense of what the supervisee wants to focus on and will ask questions to help them set the agenda, such as, "What would be useful to talk about today?" (https://pluralisticpractice.com/category/supervision/ Retrieved 6 May 2021). However, he also described how he would not shy away from an issue in supervision that feels important to focus on. This approach serves two purposes: drawing on the supervisee's strengths and the knowledge and experience of the supervisor. Creaner and Timulak (2016) suggested that a supervisor who encourages a supervisee to explore their strengths as a therapist is likely to provide "modelling for balanced self-evaluation" (p. 319). Asking questions such as, "what went well in your work with this client?" (Creaner & Timulak, 2016, p. 319) can help supervisees avoid only focusing on what they need to improve on.

Grant, Schofield and Crawford (2012) discussed how Safran and Muran (2000) suggested proficient supervisors could anticipate potential problems, engaging in early discussions "of supervisee expectations and how inevitable conflict will be handled" (p. 537). In addition, Grant et al. (2012) suggested how "highly experienced supervisors were able to demonstrate advanced capacities in maintaining (or repairing) a good supervisory alliance" (p. 537); acknowledged and reflected on their mistakes, understood the needs of different supervisees, and could be flexible to meet the needs of each situation and each supervisee.

Such flexibility is a significant feature in the pluralistic approach, with Cooper (2019) stating, "I really like the flexibility, creativity, and engagement that comes from this way of working. It feels very collaborative, dialogic, and drawing on the skills and understandings of both myself and my supervisee". (https://pluralisticpractice.com/category/supervision/ Retrieved 6 May 2021). Flexibility in pluralistic supervision is also apparent by the supervisor encouraging the supervisee to sometimes look at their work from different theoretical perspectives. Cooper suggested he would help the supervisee develop their understanding in this way and may ask, "What would be best to do here from a person-centred/psychodynamic/CBT angle?" (https://pluralisticpractice.com/category/supervision/ Retrieved 6 May 2021). At other times Cooper (2019) will remind the supervisee to include the client in any decision of how to work in therapy, exploring what the client thinks will be best for them to establish and maintain a collaborative relationship.

Pluralistic sand-tray supervision

Bainum et al., (2006) described how sand-tray therapy helps clients engage in a more profound reflective process, which may have the same benefit for therapists in supervision. Garza and Watts (2009, in Stark et al., 2011) agreed that using a sand tray in supervision helps supervisees embrace and explore their innermost thoughts and feelings.

This creative outlet is concrete, using touchable symbols that increase "reflection skills, develop awareness and insight, or conceptualise challenging cases" (Garett, 2017, p. 40). The symbolic objects empower therapists "to cope with difficulties by strengthening introspection" (Lahad, 2000, p. 15) to explore the metaphor symbolising problems like "stuckness." Like Gestalt, pluralistic sand-tray therapy facilitates exploring the internal, intrapsychic experience of the supervisee, inter-relational issues, physical processes like touch and physical sensations in response to working with the client; once explored, any insight gained, can effectively contribute to their work with their clients.

There is an assumption by various scholars that a therapist delivering sand-tray therapy with clients will use sand-tray work in their clinical supervision (Drewes & Mullen, 2008; Turner, 2005; Homeyer & Sweeney, 1998; Kwiatkowska, 1978). For example, a supervisee may need to understand their client's feeling of shame, and the supervisor may suggest they select objects to symbolise their perception of the client's shame. With the help of the supervisor and the symbolism of the objects, the supervisee can work at the "edge of awareness" (Gendlin, 1984), bringing a deeper understanding of their own perceptions and the client's thoughts and feelings. Holt et al. (2014) suggested how the physical picture in the sand can help the supervisee to observe the issue from different angles, can "illicit different responses" (p. 504) and bring a fresh perspective.

Traditional clinical supervision is predominantly restricted to verbal communication (Kwiatkowska, 1978). However, using a sand tray can help explore the supervisee's inner experience, which might not be verbally disclosed. For example, sand-tray therapy involves projective processing that can expose a therapist's personal struggle concerning an aspect of their practice. Drewes and Mullen (2008) view this non-threatening intervention as a vital aid in supervision. Luke (2008) suggested how the spontaneous, playful nature of using sand tray elicits risk-taking and produces an aspect of self, which is "authentically based rather than based on external perceptions and expectations" (p. 278).

Graham et al. (2014) research focused on exploring three creative approaches to clinical supervision and using a sand tray was one of them. They argued that this type of creative approach was less threatening than more traditional evaluative approaches to supervision, stating that it provides "a venue for deep reflection and growth" is freeing and decreases "the supervisees' defensiveness" (p. 424). The safe environment of the sand tray enables exploration; the supervisee avoids becoming hypersensitive to the evaluation process (Stark et al., 2011).

Bernard and Goodyear (1998) suggested how a sand-tray supervisor would need to be aware of adopting the different roles of consultant, teacher, and therapist. Carnes-Holt et al. (2014) described how the supervisor in the role of teacher would share their knowledge of using sand tray with clients to help the supervisee develop their skills. In addition, Drewes and Mullen (2008) argued how therapists need to have personal experience of sand-tray work before offering this way of working to clients. They suggest how this personal experience will give a "depth of understanding to use this modality effect-ively" (p. 234), which applies to supervisors also.

In pluralistic sand-tray supervision, it will also be essential to monitor and guide the supervisee to embed pluralistic principles into their sand-tray work with clients. For example, to focus on establishing a collaborative relation-ship with their clients, drawing on other methods to meet the client's goals, taking every opportunity to facilitate dialogical discussion and incorporating feedback.

Supervision practice examples

In my clinical supervision supporting the clients in the case study research, my goal for a particular session with Shirley (Fleet, 2019; Fleet et al., 2016) was to explore her feeling trapped by her anxiety, symbolised by a small wooden box with the lid closed. As I looked at the box during my supervision session, the supervisor asked, "What is in the box?" (Fleet, 2019, p. 104; Fleet et al., 2016, p. 335).

I took some moments to consider, then replied, "Her fear, her anxiety, it's trapped within her, hard to get out. She lets out some of that fear, feels some of it, but then becomes completely overwhelmed". I was then asked, "What is going on for you right now?" I described how I wanted her to escape but wondered if Shirley would ever be able to, which resulted in me feeling helpless. My supervisor's questions helped clarify how stuck I felt and to own and express my fear that I might not be able to help Shirley overcome her severe anxiety. We went on to explore my experience of feeling deskilled and concluded that I needed to stay alongside Shirley, holding on to the hope that she might break free and face her fear as the therapy progressed, easing my sense of responsibility.

By the end of therapy, Shirley had faced her fear and was managing her anxiety much more effectively; she represented her progress by placing the small wooden box in the sand but with its lid open, no longer feeling trapped.

Another object I have used in clinical supervision is a small cage, but large enough to house another small object to symbolise feeling trapped. Once again, this object helped me work on my "stuckness" with clients. Examples included clients who were depressed, anxious, and fearful and who were struggling to progress. In one supervision session, my "stuckness" was symbolised by placing a small bird in the cage with the door closed. Deeper reflection facilitated the realisation of how a dual-process was evident; the client and I both felt stuck in the process, and I was finding it difficult to hang on to hope that this client would ever progress. This was explored by a challenge from the supervisor of "okay, let's open the cage door." Once I accepted the challenge and opened the door, the question of "now what can you feel?" helped me step outside my fear. The following question of "what is the payoff from staying in the cage?" challenged me to explore and own my sense of vulnerability concerning the fear of "what if I fail and the client gave up or became suicidal?" It seemed a safer place for the client than facing their fear, and for myself as a therapist, although uncomfortable, it appeared safer than challenging a vulnerable client. This awareness helped me stay in the moment with the client rather than be concerned with "the what if?" To be fully present, moment-to-moment, helping them stay in the "now" rather than retreat to concerns of the past or future.

At other times, using the sand tray, I have used Lego bricks to build a wall around an object representing a client who kept me at a distance, no matter how I tried to help them connect and express their feelings. The supervisor challenged me by asking, "okay, that is how you see the client being stuck… what about you?" I selected a figure to represent myself and also built a wall around that object. Staying with the metaphor, we then explored what could break down those walls, helping once again to stay present and challenge the client when they were becoming distant, moving away from their feelings in successive sessions.

A supervisee and supervisor may also take a more unstructured approach when using the sand tray in pluralistic supervision. The supervisee might hold the client in their minds-eye and spontaneously create a sand display. The following questions asked by the supervisor may help with the reflective process:

- What stands out to you when you look at that scene?
- When you think of your client, is there anything missing that you could represent with an object?
- Where are you in that scene?

Supervision with a therapist new to sand-tray work

A therapist interested in delivering pluralistic sand-tray therapy may have experienced this approach during their training, attended workshops, accessed literature on pluralistic sand-tray therapy, had previously used creative ways of working in their practice with clients and now see the benefit of offering this approach to clients who are open to working that way. However, a therapist new to pluralistic sand-tray therapy will need appropriate supervision. A skilled supervisor can help prepare the therapist and develop their skills to understand both pluralistic and sand-tray processes. Before using this approach, an essential point of consideration is that the therapist needs to have a confident attitude to facilitate the client to work in this way and access supervision from a supervisor who knows about working pluralistically when using a sand tray with clients.

Summary of essential qualities and experience required of a supervisor for pluralistic sand-tray therapy

In addition, to the traditional supervision qualifications and experience, the supervisor of pluralistic sand-tray therapy will need:

* Knowledge and experience of the pluralistic approach.
  * Establishing a collaborative relationship in therapy and supervision.
  * Setting goals and expectations for therapy and supervision.
  * Establishing a culture of feedback with the supervisee's clients and in the supervisory relationship.
  * Utilising various methods of assessment and feedback (including clinical measures) in therapy and supervision.
  * Facilitating purposeful dialogue in both therapy and supervision.
  * Accepting and facilitating the benefits of drawing on other methods from various approaches to meet the client's goals.
* Knowledge and experience of sand-tray therapy/creative practice.
  * Work with symbolism and metaphor.
  * Use sand tray in supervision to support the supervisee's process.
  * To consider engaging in some personal experience of sand-tray work.
  * Feedback to help the supervisee improve their practice for future work.

Summary of the key considerations for a supervisee attending pluralistic sand-tray supervision

* To establish goals and expectations for each session.
* Materials – mobile sand tray (or supervisor's sand tray), range of objects, client's goals/expectations for therapy, client feedback, and clinical outcome measures.
* Supervisee to adopt an open and non-defensive attitude to explore the symbolism related to:
  * Client's process – verbal, nonverbal, symbolism of the objects, metaphor.
  * Supervisee's own process – perceptions, fears, assumptions, difficulties.
  * Explore the dynamics in the relationship between therapist-client and supervisee-supervisor.
  * Barriers to the process – e.g. "stuckness" in their work with the client and in supervision.

- To explore unanswered questions both regarding their work with the client and the supervisor.
- Some time spent on initial appointment (goals, tasks, and methods for therapy), clinical assessment measures (pre and post), client feedback, and if the client met their goals by the end of therapy and how this process was managed.
- Some time spent on their feedback to the supervisor and if any changes need to be discussed.
- How to improve their practice for future work.

References

Alfonsson, S., Lundgren T., & Andersson, G. (2020). Clinical supervision in cognitive behavior therapy improves therapists' competence: a single-case experimental pilot study. *Cognitive Behaviour Therapy*. 49(5), 435–438.

Bainum, C. R., Schneider, M. F., & Stone, M. H. (2006). An Adlerian model of sand-tray therapy. *Journal of Individual Psychology*, 62, 36–46.

Barber, J. P., Liese, B. S., & Abrams, M. J. (2003). Development of the cognitive therapy adherence and competence scale. *Psychotherapy Research*. 13(2), 205–221. https://doi.org/10.1093/ptr/kpg019

Beisser, A (1970). The Paradoxical Theory of Change. In J. Fagan & I Shepherds (eds.). *Gestalt Therapy Now: Theory, Techniques, and Applications*. pp. 77–80. Palo Alto, CA: Science and Behaviour Books.

Bernard, J., & Goodyear, R. (1998). *Fundamentals of Clinical Supervision*. Boston: Allyn & Bacon.

Borders, L. D. (2014). Best practices in clinical supervision: Another step in delineating effective supervision practice. *American Journal of Psychotherapy*, 68(2), 151–162.

Bordin E. S. (1983). A working alliance based model of supervision. *Counseling Psychologist*. 11, 35–42.

Brown, B. www.pinterest.at/ Retrieved 26 April 2021.

Callifronas, M. D., & Brock, S. (2017). A person-centred view of the aim, goals and tasks in clinical supervision: Proposals on topics for experiential learning. *British Journal of Medicine & Medical Research*. 19(8): 1–12. Article no. BJMMR.29507

Carnes-Holt, K., Meany-Walen, K., & Felton, A. (2014). Utilizing sandtray within the discrimination model of counselor supervision. *Journal of Creativity in Mental Health*. 9, 497–510.

Carson, D. K., & Becker, K. W. (2004). When lightning strikes: Reexamining creativity in psychotherapy. *Journal of Counseling and Development*. 22 (1), 111–115.

Casado-Kehoe, M., & Ybañez, K. (2011). Clinical Supervision. In Suzanne Degges-White and Nancy L. Davis. Integrating the Expressive Arts Into Counseling Practice Theory-Based Interventions. Chapter 12. New York: Springer Publishing Company, LLC.

Cooper, M. (2019). Supervising from a Pluralistic Perspective. June 13, 2019. https://pluralisticpractice.com/category/supervision/ Retrieved 30 April, 2021.

Creaner, M., & Timulak, L. (2016). Supervision in Pluralistic Counselling and Psychotherapy. In Mick Cooper and Windy Dryden's (Eds.). *The Handbook of Pluralistic Counselling and Psychotherapy*. Chapter 25, pp. 314–325. London: Sage.

Drewes, A. A., & Mullen, J, A. (2008). *Supervision Can Be Playful: Techniques for Child and Play Therapist Supervision.* New York: Jason Aronson.

Dryden, W., & Thorne, B. (1991). *Training and supervision for counselling in action.* London: Sage Publications.

Ellis, M. V. (1991). Critical incidents in clinical supervision and in supervisor supervision: Assessing supervisory issues. *Journal of Counseling Psychology*, 38(3), 342–349. https://doi.org/10.1037/0022-0167.38.3.342

Fleet, D, Burton, A., Reeves, A., & DasGupta, M. P. (2016). A case for taking the dual role of counsellor-researcher in qualitative research. *Qualitative Research in Psychology*, 13(4), 328–346.

Fleet, D. (2019). *Transformation hidden in the sand: developing a theoretical framework using a sand-tray intervention with adult clients.* Doctoral thesis. Staffordshire University. Stoke-on-Trent. Available from Ethos STORE – Staffordshire Online Repository. https://eprints.staffs.ac.uk/id/eprint/5763

Garrett, M. (2017). Enhancing counselor supervision with sandtray interventions. *Journal of Higher Education Theory and Practice*, 17(5), 39–44.

Garza, Y., & Watts, R. E. (2009). Sandtray: Whispers from the soul, crafted in the sand. Preconference workshop presented at the meeting of the Texas Counseling Association, Dallas, TX. In Marcella D. Stark, Rebecca K. Frels & Yvonne Garza (2011): The Use of Sandtray in Solution-Focused Supervision. *The Clinical Supervisor,* 30:2, 277–290 http://dx.doi.org/10.1080/07325223.2011.621869

Gendlin, E. T. (1984). *The Client's Client: The Edge of Awareness.* In R.L. Levant & J.M. Shlien (Eds.), *Client-Centered Therapy and the Person-Centered Approach. New Directions in Theory, Research and Practice.* New York: Praeger.

Gorden, P. K. (2012). Ten steps to cognitive behavioural supervision. *The Cognitive Behaviour Therapist*, 5(4), 71–82. American Psychological Association. doi.org/10.1017/S1754470X12000050

Graham, M. A., Scholl, M. B., Smith-Adcock, S., & Wittmann, E. (2014) Three creative approaches to counseling supervision, *Journal of Creativity in Mental Health.* 9(3), 415–426. DOI: 10.1080/15401383.2014.899482

Grant, J., Schofield, M. J., & Crawford, S. (2012). Managing difficulties in supervision: Supervisors' perspectives. *Journal of Counseling Psychology.* 59(4), 528–541. American Psychological Association.

Hackney, H., & Goodyear, R. K. (1984). Carl Rogers's Client-Centered Approach to Supervision. In R. F. Levant & J. M. Shlien (Eds.), *Client Centered Therapy and the Person Centered Approach: New Directions in Theory, Research, and Practice* Chapter 14, pp. 278–296. Westport: Praeger Publishers.

Holt, K. C., Meany-Walen, K. & Felton, A. (2014). Utilizing sandtray within the discrimination model of counselor supervision. *Journal of Creativity in Mental Health*, 2(1), 13–33.

Homeyer, L., & Sweeney, D. (1998). *Sandtray: A Practical Manual.* Canyon Lake. TX: Lindan Press.

Houston, K. T. (2013). *Speech-Language Pathology.* San Diego, CA: Plural Publishing.

Kwiatkowska, H. (1978). *Family Therapy and Evaluation Through Art.* Springfield, IL: Charles C. Thomas.

Ladany, N. (2004). Psychotherapy supervision: What lies beneath. *Psychotherapy Research*, 14, 1–19. doi:10.1093/ptr/kph001

Lahad, M. (2000). *Creative Supervision: The Use of Expressive Arts Methods in Super-Vision and Self-Supervision*. Philadelphia, PA: Jessica Kingsley Publishers.

Lambers, E. (2013). Supervision. In M. Cooper, M. O'Hara, P. F. Schmid, & A. C. Bohart (Eds.), *The Handbook of Person-Centred Psychotherapy & Counselling* (2nd ed.) (pp. 453–467). London, England: Palgrave Macmillan.

Lombardo, C., Milne, D., & Procter, R. (2009). Getting to the heart of clinical supervision: a theoretical review of the role of emotions in professional development. *Behavioural and Cognitive Psychotherapy* 37, 207–219.

Luke, M. (2008). Supervision: Models, principles, and process issues. In A. A. Drewes, & J. A. Mullen (Eds.), *Supervision Can Be Playful: Techniques for Child and Play Therapist Supervisors* (pp. 7–25). New York: Jason Aronson.

Turner, B. A. (2005). *The Handbook of Sandplay Therapy*. California, USA: Temenos Press.

McLeod, J. (2018). *Pluralistic Therapy; Distinctive Features*. London: Routledge, Taylor and Francis Group.

Mearns, D. (1997). *Person-Centred Counselling Training*. London, England: Sage.

Milne, D., Reiser, R., Aylott, H., Dunkerley, C., Fitzpatrick, H., & Wharton, S. (2010). The systematic review as an empirical approach to improving CBT supervision. *International Journal of Cognitive Therapy*. 3, 278–294.

Milne, D. L., & Watkins C. E. (2014). Defining and Understanding Clinical Supervision: A Functional Approach. In: Watkins C. E, Milne D. L. (Eds.). *The Wiley International Handbook of Clinical Supervision*. Chichester: Wiley. pp. 3–19.

Muse, K., McManus, F., Rakovshik, S., & Thwaites, R. (2017). Development and psychometric evaluation of the Assessment of Core CBT Skills (ACCS): An observation-based tool for assessing cognitive behavioral therapy competence. *Psychological Assessment*, 29(5), 542. https://doi.org/10.1037/pas0000372

Patterson, C. H. (1983). A client-Centered Approach to Supervision. *The Counseling Psychologist*. 11(1), 21–25. https://doi.org/10.1177/0011000083111005

Ramos-Sánchez, L., Esnil, E., Goodwin, A., Riggs, S., Touster, L. O., Wright, L. K., & Rodolfa, E. (2002). Negative supervisory events: Effects on supervision and supervisory alliance. Professional Psychology: *Research and Practice*. 33(2), 197–202. doi:10.1037/0735-7028.33.2.197

Rice, L. N. (1980). A client-centered approach to the supervision of psychotherapy. *Psychotherapy supervision: Theory, research and practice*. 136–147.

Sommers-Flanagan, J., & Sommers-Flanagan, R. (2012). *Counseling & Psychotherapy Theories in Context and Practice: Skills, Strategies, and Techniques*. 2nd edition. John Wiley & Sons.

Stark, M. D., & Frels, R. K., & Garza, Y. (2011). The use of sandtray in solution-focused supervision. *The Clinical Supervisor*. 30, 277–290. doi: 10.1080/07325223.2011.621869

Sweeney, J., & Creaner, M. (2014). What's not being said? Recollections of nondisclosure in clinical supervision while in training. *British Journal of Guidance & Counselling*. 42(2), 211–224.

Tally, L. P., & Jones, L. (2019) Person-centered supervision: A realistic approach to practice within counselor education. *Teaching and Supervision in Counseling*. 1(2), 20–30.

Villas-Boas Bowen, M. C. (2002). Personality Differences and Person-Centered Supervision. In D. J. Cain (Ed.), *Classics in the Person-Centered Approach.* (pp. 92–103). Ross-on-Wye, UK: PCCS Books.

Watkins, E., & Milne, D. L. (2014*). The Wiley International Handbook of Clinical Supervision*, First Edition. Edited by C. Edward Watkins, Jr. and Derek L. Milne. Chichester, West Sussex: John Wiley & Sons, Ltd.

Chapter 12

Drawing on other theoretical orientations in pluralistic sand-tray therapy

If you have knowledge, let others light their candles in it

(Margaret Fuller. [1810–1850] https://in.pinterest.com)

Throughout this book, the drawing on other methods from various orientations has been emphasised, which can help clients meet their goals and expectations in pluralistic therapy. The strengths and opinions of the client and the knowledge and experience of the therapist to establish a collaborative relationship are also significant features in pluralistic therapy. This chapter will explain how to draw on other orientations and incorporate such methods into pluralistic sand-tray therapy.

Humanistic

The PCT approach (Rogers, 1957; 1961) and Gestalt therapy (Perls, 1973) are two dominant orientations within humanistic psychotherapy. Although there are some differences in terms of their underpinning philosophies and therapeutic approach, they do "share a common humanistic foundation" that "people are unique, greater than the sum of their parts" (Hanley et al., 2016, p. 95). They also agree that a person has the potential for constructive growth and can make choices in their lives (Bugental, 1964). Pluralistic sand-tray therapy is also fundamentally built on these humanistic assumptions; the client's uniqueness, potential growth, and ability to exercise a significant capacity for choice. The client is encouraged to contribute to any decisions made throughout the therapy process; these aspects function as building blocks to establish a collaborative therapeutic relationship.

Hanley et al. (2016) discussed how PCT, founded by Carl Rogers, is "the most common variant that comes under the humanistic therapy umbrella" (p. 96).

However, Sanders (2004/2012) has described how PCT is not homogenous, being made up of a range of stances he described as "tribes."

DOI: 10.4324/9781003158707-12

Sanders views PCT as incorporating tribes such as classical client-centred therapy, focusing-orientated therapy, experiential person-centred therapy, emotion-focused therapy, and existentially informed person-centred therapy (2012, p. 247) in his pivotal book "The Tribes of the Person-Centred Nation."

Classical person-centred therapy

Merry (2004) summarises classical PCT with "the theory of actualisation is regarded as the sole motivation for human behaviour, growth, change and development" (pp. 42–43), and the underpinning theory of PCT is based on this assumption. Rogers (1951) understanding of the actualising tendency is how a person will continue to strive to fulfil their potential. Later, Rogers suggested how "the Actualising Tendency can, of course, be thwarted or warped, but it cannot be destroyed without destroying the organism" (1980, p. 118). However, in a safe and accepting relationship, constructive development will occur (Merry, 2004).

The therapist adopts a non-directive attitude, respecting the client's capacity for change and their psychological determination based on the argument that any effort to direct therapy undermines the client as expert of their own process (Merry, 2004). Techniques and strategies are not part of classical PCT; instead, the core belief is that "the PCT relationship is the therapy" (Merry, 2004, p. 42).

Rogers approach was phenomenological, based on the assumption that to understand a person's feelings and behaviour, it is necessary to understand their subjective experience and how they perceive the world in which they live (Rogers 1961). Pluralistic sand-tray therapy also works with the client's phenomenological experience. The view is that each client is unique and the symbolic objects used in the process facilitate them to explore their own inner-experience and their perceptions of the world.

Merry (2004) also postulated that the therapeutic relationship where Rogers six "necessary and sufficient conditions of therapeutic personality change" provides the corrective environment for a client's psychological damage. "Three of the six conditions have been identified as most important, or at least have received the most attention, becoming known as the core conditions" (Merry, 2004, p. 31); empathic understanding, congruence, and unconditional positive regard (UPR).

Merry (2004) described empathic understanding as staying alongside the client's internal frame of reference, grasping how they see the world and with the therapist setting aside their own assumptions as far as possible. In pluralistic sand-tray therapy, the therapist will endeavour to see the client's world represented in the sand tray and verbally communicate this in their responses to the client. By "stepping into the client's shoes," they communicate, I see your world, hear your thoughts, and acknowledge your feelings, establishing a safe and protected space for the client to explore.

UPR concerns the non-judgemental and accepting attitude of the therapist concerning the client's experience. It is not about approving destructive behaviour of the client but described by Merry (2004) as a "consistent acceptance" and "non-possessive caring" (p. 36). In pluralistic sand-tray therapy, UPR is particularly relevant in acknowledging and respecting the client's interpretation of the objects selected to represent their experience. The therapist will need to stay alongside the client and avoid imposing their interpretations of the objects. Any shift to the therapist's frame of reference could risk a rupture in the relationship and result in the client disengaging. Each object will have a specific meaning for an individual client, and the therapist will need to stay close to that symbolism so the client feels understood and respected. For example, a lion may represent a threat to one client, yet protection to another.

UPR can also be offered to the client by acknowledging how they work with the sand tray, encouraging them to continue to engage, giving reassurance that there is no right way or wrong way to work with the objects in the sand. Furthermore, UPR is relevant by respecting and facilitating the client's input concerning their goals and expectations for therapy and the tasks and methods. Any decision made will be collaborative, involving two-way dialogue, with the therapist asking the client, "what do you think might work best for you?"

Congruency, sometimes described as being genuine and real corresponds to a therapist who is a self-aware person; "aware of their feelings, emotions and sensations without blocking them off" (Merry, 2004, p. 35), and their behaviour in the therapeutic relationship is consistent with their inner feelings and emotions.

Congruency in pluralistic sand-tray therapy involves the therapist being real when establishing a collaborative relationship with the client. The therapist draws on their knowledge and experience, sharing this with the client when appropriate, without adopting the expert stance. The aim is to facilitate a dialogical conversation with the client bringing their own opinion when considering what they think might work best for them. Congruency will also involve the therapist sharing their response to an action, thought or feeling communicated by the client when appropriate. For example, the client might be working with their grief concerning bereavement and may have symbolised their loss by selecting an object to represent the deceased and places the object outside the sand tray. The therapist might respond, "and they've gone, no seeing, no touching, no holding them, I feel a real sadness as you removed that." Such a reflection might help the client connect more deeply with their sadness and loss.

Focusing-orientated therapy

Purton (2012) describes how focusing-orientated therapy (FOT) developed from Eugene Gendlin's philosophy of "how our lived experiences are related to the way we talk about them" (p. 47). Like PCT and psychodynamic therapy, FOT aims to help clients express themselves authentically (Purton, 2012). PCT helps the client become more congruent, psychodynamic aims to make unconscious experience conscious and FOT aims to help the client become more authentic so that they can "express themselves more adequately, to live more fully" (Purton, 2012, p. 48).

Gendlin (1969) outlined focusing as a process that brings awareness into the body, achieving a felt sense in words or images. Purton (2012) discussed how Gendlin argued how clients make good progress when they "do something different in their sessions" (p. 53) rather than simply reporting their experience and become submerged in their feelings. For example, a client who pauses after some self-disclosure to reflect on what they have communicated helps them find a new perspective and a novel way to express their experience (Gendlin, 1996), often demonstrating surprise or insight.

Gendlin (1996) refers to a case study where the client focused on her problematic relationship with her husband and described how she wanted to put him into a cello case and remould him. The therapist suggested the client sense that a little longer; after a pause and some reflection, she realised that although she wanted to put him away at that time in a safe place, she did want him back.

Similarly, in the case study (Fleet, 2019), Grace paused and reflected on the upturned spider object in the sand representing her husband. He was a heavy alcohol drinker, and she expressed surprise when she related the dead spider to the death of her relationship (Chapter 4). Her felt sense, symbolised by the spider object, helped her find the words to express the probability that her relationship with her husband was over.

In FOT, the therapist may use a procedure such as two-chair work to help the client gain a fresh response to their situation, helping them "express things that they have not been able to express" (Purton, 2012, p. 66). The therapist will then help the client explore how they feel after the procedure to ascertain a difference in how they perceive the situation.

Similarly, in the case study (Fleet, 2019), Shirley was able to talk about something she had been struggling to express by working with the objects of a closed-box and religious figures. She was able to speak out loud a question she had not been able to say before, of "is God real?" (Chapter 4). Once spoken, her body became relaxed, and she sat back in the chair. Her outlook was different as she had expressed a part of herself she had kept hidden. Purton (2012) advises therapists to ask the question, "has what was done helped them to move on a little, to become more 'themself'?" (p. 66); this seemed to be the case for Shirley. In FOT, the therapist will help the client explore how specific things are different by using active listening and reflecting.

In pluralistic sand-tray therapy, this process will involve purposeful questions.

Experiential person-centred therapy

In PCE "the therapist listens, and keeps checking with the client, and the client in turn checks with their experiential flow within." (Baker, 2012, p.77). This approach involves the client's non-verbal behaviour in addition to the words they use to express themselves (Baker, 2012). PCET acknowledges Gendlin's (1984) edge of awareness work where the felt sense at the border zone can become explicit and recognised by the client, patiently allowing personal meaning to emerge.

In summary, PCET draws on the client's intrapsychic/interpersonal experience and process work that involves how the client is with their feelings and how they are handling their feelings. Baker (2012) described, "how the client presents is the key" (p. 82), and as the therapist listens to their verbal and visual cues, so the client feels deeply heard, they become closer to the client's flow of experience and respond sensitively to the client who may be experiencing inner conflict.

Working with a client's intrapsychic and interpersonal experience are also significant features of pluralistic sand-tray therapy. Rogers (1951) referred to the term "incongruence" to explain psychological disturbance; Freeth (2007) discussed McMillan's (2004) notion of "intrapersonal congruence," adapting this to "intrapersonal incongruence" and explaining this as "a disturbance within individuals" (p.32). The individual might distort a disturbing emotional experience, which is then only partially symbolised. McMillan (2004) refers to the example of when a person believes they are a failure; yet when they succeed at something, puts this down to good luck.

Pluralistic sand-tray therapy aids the exploration of such inner conflict and aims to help the client experience a phenomenological shift concerning their issues, helping them reduce their psychological and emotional distress.

Baker (2012) also suggested how "experiential therapists do not do anything to the client" (p. 91). Instead, the therapist continues checking out their understandings with the client, firmly attuned to them. Once again, a therapist delivering pluralistic sand-tray work will facilitate purposeful discussion throughout therapy, which also involves checking with the client that they feel understood and contributing to the therapeutic process.

In PCET, the client is facilitated to "access their inner wisdom in a more pro-active way" (p. 93) than for classical PCT; the therapist pays close attention to the client's behaviour "and how they process their experiences" (Baker, 2012, p. 93). In addition, the PCET therapist will actively challenge the client to work at the edge of awareness and have goals to help their clients to become "more in touch with their inner experiencing and to honour their pre-verbal felt senses" (Baker, 2012, p. 94).

Edge of awareness experience is a significant element of pluralistic sand-tray therapy with regard to working with the symbolic objects representing the client's experience. The symbolic process aids edge of awareness exploration and facilitates the client to make explicit the implicit as they find their "right" words to communicate their felt sense.

Emotion-focused therapy

Elliott (2012) described how emotion-focused therapy (EFT), sometimes described as process-experiential therapy, is an approach that actively integrates Gestalt and other humanistic approaches, framed by the person-centred relationship (Greenberg et al., 2004). The main emphasis of EFT is to establish a therapeutic relationship based on a genuine, empathic, and prizing attitude and adopt an "active, task-focused process-guiding style of Gestalt therapy (Perls, 1969) and focusing (Gendlin, 1981), among others" (Elliott, 2012, p. 103). Tasks can include two-chair dialogue (Greenberg, 1979), which helps a client work through a conflictual experience, two chair enactment to work on self-interruption linked to emotional blocking or empty-chair work, linked to unfinished business (Elliott, 2012).

This way of working can be adopted in pluralistic sand-tray therapy, with the sand tray separated into two parts and dialogue facilitated between the two opposing elements (people or parts of self) involved in the conflict.

Similarly, the client can represent their "unfinished business" with objects and speak out loud something they did not get the chance or decided not to say (Chapter 6: Speaking the unspoken/unfinished business).

Existentially informed person-centred therapy

Cooper (2012) discussed some of the concepts within the existential view of the person, making his first point that existential theory emphasises the uniqueness of each human being similar to classical client-centred theory.

Pluralistic sand-tray therapy also views the individual as unique, so it is vital to establish a collaborative relationship that draws on the client's personal strengths and the knowledge and experience of the therapist.

Although Cooper acknowledges the similar view between Client-centered therapy (CCT) and the existential approach, he points out that CCT assumes that every individual is motivated towards growth in relation to their actualising tendency, which is questioned from an existential stance, arguing that some people might be inclined towards self-destruction.

Other similarities between existential informed PCT and CCT include understanding the client from a subjective, lived-experience stance, viewing psychological disturbance related to distortion or denial of experiences. Both stances do not use therapy techniques and accept the client, whatever their behaviour (Cooper, 2012).

In terms of pluralistic sand-tray therapy, some psychological problems are viewed as a distortion or denial of lived experience and acknowledge some of that disturbance due to unconscious conflict, which can be accessed via the symbolic sand-tray process. However, some problems may be due to another's behaviour the client is in a relationship with or connected to the wider world.

Cooper (2012) discussed the differences between the PCT and Existential PCT, describing how the existential approach places more emphasis on the choice and agency of the client regarding change and "less emphasis on the client's inherent tendency to find the answers that are right for them" (p. 158), with the therapist sometimes taking a directive approach.

Pluralistic sand-tray therapy agrees with this stance and encourages clients to contribute to purposeful discussion on goal setting, any decision made about how to work in therapy and feedback. In addition, distortion and denial are understood to derive from internal and external sources, helping clients come to terms with limitations and discomfort, viewing these experiences as part of the human condition rather than surpassing them (Cooper, 2012). In pluralistic sand-tray therapy, helping clients come to terms with their limitations and discomfort is led by the client. For example, in the case study (Fleet, 2019), Anne, who had a severe accident to her leg, eventually moved to a state of accepting her limitations and how her life needed to change because of her restrictions. Once she had expressed her anger, fear, and sadness of losing her full capability to run, dance, and go on long walks, this acceptance occurred. Near the end of therapy, it was vital to acknowledge her new perception that she could still be happy and could engage in some activities but with restrictions.

Finally, Cooper (2012) discussed how a therapist who works from an existential PCT stance would adopt a less individualistic focus, facilitating "clients to consider the needs, feelings and demands of others, rather than just their own" (p. 158). Returning to Anne once again, in her pluralistic sand-tray therapy, she was challenged in a similar way to consider how her husband might be feeling by acknowledging how she always tries to get her own way. This shift resulted in Anne giving him some consideration, and she shared how she needed to take a fairer stance with him and not always try and get her way in her relationship.

Gestalt therapy

Stevens (2004) used sand tray as part of a gestalt approach, mainly with adult clients and viewed this way of working as a "simple form of experimentation" (p. 18). The gestalt therapist using sand tray does not interpret the client's experience but is not a passive observer either (Stevens, 2004). Like pluralistic sand-tray therapy, the gestalt relationship is a dialogical encounter that explores the client's experience beyond the limitations of words alone (Stevens, 2004). Stevens (2004) stated how gestalt therapy is about "the contacting process itself" (p. 5) and being aware of what is emerging in the here and now. As the client becomes interested, they gain energy "until contact is heightened, awareness brightened, behaviour energized" (Perls et al., 1994, p. 232). The aim to help the client become fully present in the moment, letting go of being preoccupied with what has happened in the past and worrying about their future.

Stevens (2004) advocates how free creative expression by the client using sand tray is essential, as each client is unique and will use the sand tray in their own way; therefore, any attempt to establish a rigid formula will be unhelpful. She also suggests that she was not attempting to inform others of "how to do sand-tray therapy, just as no one has told me how to do it" (2004, p. 7) – arguing that observing other therapists and reading the literature helps therapists to integrate this way of working into their therapeutic approach.

The pluralistic sand-tray approach agrees that each client will want to work with the sand tray in their own way, and there is a need for a collaborative relationship to meet their needs and goals. Attending workshops on sand-tray therapy, taking part in seminars based on sand-tray work during counsellor training and reading the literature on sand-tray therapy can help build confidence for the therapist, aiming to integrate sand-tray work into their approach. However, it is crucial to keep in mind that each client is unique, and any intervention during a sand-tray session needs to be based on the client's frame of reference and their process during therapy. This stance directly conflicts with the Jungian (Kalff, 1980) and Homeyer and Sweeney's (2011) eclectic approach, emphasising specific sand-tray training requirements.

Stevens (2004) views sand tray as an experiment, offering something new in order to gain understanding when a client is experiencing a block to being fully present and engaged in therapy. Sometimes adult clients can demonstrate resistance to experiencing their feelings or becoming involved in the creative process, having a tendency to intellectualise. She (2004) argued how the symbolic processes of sand-tray work could bypass such resistances.

The gestalt therapist using a sand tray will adopt a more active role than a Jungian or PCT therapist. Stevens (2004) suggests how the gestalt therapist will be curious about the sand display and ask questions, becoming engaged in the client's process. At times during pluralistic sand-tray therapy, the therapist will also ask Socratic questions to help facilitate edge of awareness and unconscious processing. In addition, therapists questions made at an appropriate time are helpful, encouraging the client to engage in purposeful discussion during therapy.

Cognitive behavioural therapy

Boucher (2016, p. 108) discusses how CBT developed through the work of a number of scholars, including "Albert Ellis's rational-emotive therapy (1962) and Aaron Beck's cognitive therapy (Beck, 1964; Beck et al., 1979)". Today CBT is one of the main psychotherapeutic approaches in existence and is approved by the National Health Service and backed by the National Institute for Health and Excellence [NICE] (Boucher, 2016).

Contemporary CBT incorporates several approaches, including compassion-focused therapy (Gilbert, 2005), schema therapy, (Young et al., 2003) and mindfulness-based cognitive therapy (Segal et al., 2002), and all incorporate the integration between behavioural and cognitive processes (Boucher, 2016). Furthermore, Boucher (2016) suggests that the practice of CBT draws on humanistic principles by offering the core conditions and functions collaboratively within the working alliance.

The concept of distorted thinking as a cause of psychological and emotional distress is a significant feature of CBT. Boyes (2008) stated how such "thoughts distort our thinking in a way that causes us to expect the worst and to feel unpleasant emotions" (p. 26). Boyes (2008) described how CBT highlight various types of distorted thinking including, all or nothing thinking, overgeneralisation, mind reading, fortune telling, catastrophising, labelling, and irrational "should," "must," "ought to," "have to" statements, leading to distress.

In CBT, the aim is to identify the negative thought and challenge this by helping the client seek evidence that contradicts the distorted thinking. At times, scales are used to give a sense of perspective. Scaling involves the client helped to rate their issue on a numerical scale from 1–10, with 1 being the least severe and 10 being the most. These scale positions are based on the client's perceptions and can help them take ownership of their treatment goals and progress (Berg & de Shazer, 1993).

Scaling can help lessen the intense emotional tone in the client's communication when identifying themselves away from the extreme ends of the scale.

Activity worksheets involving homework, also used in CBT, help the client work on their distorted thinking patterns between sessions.

Pluralistic sand-tray therapy can draw on the concept of distorted thinking when applicable to a client. For example, all or nothing thinking can be explored using the sand tray. The therapist could suggest the client splits the sand tray into three and select objects to represent the polar opposite thinking concerning an issue. The client is then helped to explore these negative patterns and is aided to express the feelings as a result of the negative thoughts. Once the client has been helped to explore these two positions, they can be challenged to select an object to represent the middle ground.

A specific example could involve a client's perfectionism, and the tray is likely to resemble perfection VS failure related to the client's experience. The perfection side of the tray is likely to be linked to the pressure of impossible expectations and the failure side to feelings of inadequacy. The middle ground linked more to self-acceptance could involve a new appreciation that the client is neither a complete failure nor a perfect person, and "good enough" might become the new goal.

Solution-focused therapy

de Shazer et al. (1986) are acknowledged to have developed solution-focused therapy (SFT). Further research (Berg, 1994; de Shazer, 1994; Corcoran &

Pillai, 2007; Kim, 2008) has expanded the understanding of SFT. Key features include focusing on the client's goals, finding exceptions to the problem, and drawing the client's strengths and resources. SFT uses various tools to facilitate the client in therapy, including the miracle question (de Shazer,1985/1988). This strategy helps the client visualise how the future would be if the problem were no longer present.

For example, the client is asked, "If you woke up tomorrow, and a miracle happened so that you no longer felt inadequate/angry/jealous (specific to the client's experience), what would be different? What would be the first sign that the miracle had happened?" The question is asked sensitively and respectfully, paying close attention to the client's body language, and with the therapist remaining silent to enable the client time to reflect.

SFT also uses the tools of CBT scaling (Berg, 1994) and coping questions. Coping questions (de Shazer et al., 1986) are designed to identify how the client has managed to cope despite the adversity they face, which the client is unaware of. An example of a coping question could be, "How do you manage to keep going every day when there seems to be no hope?" Coping questions helps clients to identify their inner resources and strengths they had not realised they had.

In contrast to the psychodynamic approach, which views a client's past and childhood experience as highly significant is not the case with SFT. Therefore, SFT does not gather a detailed history of the client as a requirement; instead, the present and the future are the focus for this approach (de Shazer et al., 1986).

SFT takes a similar view to PCT that the client is the key to bringing change, but in SFT, there is a focus on solutions rather than facilitating the client to become more congruent. For example, Mearns and Thorne (1999), from a PCT standpoint, stated how progress would involve the client being able to express their feelings in "a straightforward, accurate way rather than hiding or disguising them" (Mearns & Thorne, 1999, p. 97).

SFT is usually short-term and, at times, can be delivered in a single session.

This exceptionally short-term therapy has been criticised; Stalker et al. (1999) argue how such brief therapy can be less effective for clients with severe problems.

Taylor (2009) suggested how the similarities between SFT and sand-tray therapy presents the opportunity to integrate the two approaches, producing an "empowering and brief experiential therapeutic journey" (p. 56) for clients.

The advantages of the therapist taking an observer role and, at times, taking a more active role is beneficial and not mutually exclusive (Taylor, 2009). An example concerns the use of the CBT miracle question using sand tray; the client is asked to select objects to symbolise their response, and then the therapist observes the clients non-verbal behaviour, as well as the chosen objects and where they were placed in the sand to help the client focus on solutions (Taylor, 2009).

However, Homeyer and Sweeney (2011) suggest that SFT interventions should not be used too early in therapy until sufficient therapeutic safety exists. Otherwise, the intervention might be detrimental and intrusive for the client. For example, clients who have experienced trauma may be closed down if asked such questions too early.

In pluralistic sand-tray therapy focusing on the client's goals, finding exceptions to the problem, and drawing the client's strengths and resources are compatible with SFT. The miracle question and coping questions can be incorporated by using the symbolic objects as Taylor (2009) suggests, but the impetus for such interventions will emerge from the client's process and frame of reference.

If the client is at a stage where they are exploring and expressing their deep emotions, then the pluralistic therapist will facilitate that process and not jump to seeking solutions. Any method adopted is agreed upon collaboratively between the therapist and the client.

Compassion-focused therapy

Compassion-focused therapy (CFT) was developed by Paul Gilbert (2009a; 2010), drawing on various theories, including evolutionary psychology, biology, Buddhist thinking, Jungian archetype theory, and neuroscience.

"Gilbert (1989, 1995, 2005b, 2009a) combined archetype theory with modern evolutionary, social and development psychology" (Gilbert 2010, p. 22). He argued how people have "social mentalities" which influence them to seek out and form specific relationships, including those, which are "sexual, tribal, dominant-subordinate, caring or-cared for" (Gilbert 2010, p. 22). For example, Gilbert (2010) describes how a person in the caregiving mentality will demonstrate concern for another and behave in a manner to attend to their needs. However, when in a care-seeking mentality, they will seek others who can provide the support and care they need.

When a person is in a competitive mentality, they will compare themselves to others, be in a state of winner-loser, and behave so that they try harder or give up. If they win, they are likely to feel good, but if they lose, they may feel defeated, angry, or envious and turn off any empathic thoughts and feelings towards the other (Gilbert, 2010).

Gilbert's (2010) concept of the "tricky brain" suggests how human brains are incredibly complex, and although they "can do amazing things" (p. 17), there are trade-offs. The cognitive capacities of "imagining, anticipating and ruminating" can be problematic as Gilbert stated, "We still have old brain emotions and motives" (Gilbert, 2010, p. 17). He uses the analogy of a zebra running away from a lion; if the zebra escapes, it will settle quickly. However, a person chased by a lion is likely to be traumatised and, even if they escape, would be preoccupied with the "what if?" They might also experience images of being eaten alive. Therefore, although the complex brain has benefits such as problem-solving, the human capacity for reflection can also lead to psychological problems. For example, a person who experiences anxiety may ruminate over a specific fear, such as something bad will happen to one of their family. Someone who is depressed may obsess that they are not good enough and will always fail.

Gilbert and Irons (2005) argued that self-criticism, self-disliking, self-hating, and shame were pervasive problems in mental health. Shame and self-criticism can have a seriously detrimental impact on an individual's emotional state and well-being.

People with a strong inner-critic will often experience a sense of hopelessness that may lead to depression (Whelton & Greenberg, 2005). Gilbert suggests how CFT acknowledges the emotions of "disappointment, frustration, anger or contempt" (2014, p. 31), viewing them as defensive emotions and part of the threat system. Also, perceiving oneself as incompetent or ugly is associated with the threat of shame and will most likely result in the person feeling disconnected, unloved, unwanted, and often defenceless (Gilbert, 2007; Gilbert & Irons, 2005). CFT helps the client recognise the threats that produce self-hatred and direct compassion to those fears and emotions that Gilbert described as sitting "behind the critic" (2014, p. 32).

Sometimes these emotions and fears may be related to memories of past experience when the person felt vulnerable or rejected, and by focusing on those emotional memories, they can be re-scripted by directing compassion to them. Gilbert suggests that this process is often associated with grief, and the client is helped to move through the process of loss.

According to Gilbert, the central concern for CFT is compassionate mind training involving the client working "with experiences of inner warmth, safeness and soothing via compassion and self-compassion" (2009b, p. 199).

Clients are helped to perceive their difficulties in compassionate ways to experience safety and warmth towards themselves and others (Kolts, 2016). CFT will also help the client by providing effective tools to manage challenging experiences associated with emotions. There are numerous CFT exercises established by Gilbert and other scholars of CFT facilitated in therapy; then, once the client feels confident, they can be practised outside of therapy in their own time. For example, soothing rhythm breathing (Gilbert www.compassionatemind.co.uk Retrieved 19 May 2021) is a step-by-step guide, helping clients gently focus on their breathing, bodily sensations and helps them stay tuned to the moment. This relaxation technique, when practised regularly, can be beneficial, reminding the client to avoid becoming preoccupied with past or future worries or concerns. Another CFT exercise can involve a relaxation exercise where the client is helped to create a calm, safe, and peaceful space within.

This exercise involves imagination; the safe place might be in a forest, near the ocean or recreate a personal memory of somewhere they felt safe and cared for. It is crucial to help the client engage their senses of sight, touch, sound, and smell to bring joy and pleasure, helping them establish an emotional connection. Other exercises will focus on extending compassion to other people.

In pluralistic sand-tray therapy, some elements of CFT can be used to help meet the client's goals and expectations of therapy. For example, the soothing rhythm exercise and creating a safe space can be facilitated, the client then selects objects to represent how they feel once the exercise is complete. The sand display is a physical picture that they can see and touch, symbolising their emotional connection to the relaxation technique. Transforming the imagined safe space to a physical representation in the sand, which can be photographed, can bring a richer experience for the client.

Schema therapy

Schema therapy was initially "developed by Young (1990) for the treatment of personality dysfunction" (Carter et al., 2013, p. 500), based on his argument that traditional CBT was less effective with such clients. Schema therapy used for complex, chronic psychological issues, including personality disorders, is increasingly being used by therapists working with depressed clients (Carter et al., 2013).

Young et al. (2003) describe how schema therapy is an integrative approach drawing on CBT, object relations theory (psychoanalytic), attachment theory, and gestalt therapy. While CBT examines the relationships between thoughts, feelings and behaviours, and changing automatic thoughts, schema therapy aims to weaken and adapt maladaptive schemas established in childhood to rectify past emotional disturbances and change long-term patterns, which have become established in adulthood.

A schema is a unit of knowledge, and new information, perceptions, and understanding are assimilated into existing schemas (Piaget, 1952). Young et al. (2003) described how the term schema "refers to an early maladaptive schema" (p. 7), which are dysfunctional patterns "of memories, emotions and physical sensations" persisting in adulthood. Farrell et al. (2014) described, "when schemas are activated, modes are triggered" (p. 6); modes corresponding to the emotions and behaviours a person experiences related to the activated schema.

For example, a child growing up in an abusive environment may have a self-schema of "I am worthless, unlovable and bad" and is likely to experience emotions such as sadness, anger, shame and behaviour like avoiding social interaction, low self-esteem, and a lack of confidence. Some may project their anger onto other people or engage in intentional self-harm, turning their anger inwards. If these patterns are persistent over time, the person may become chronically depressed.

A wide range of experiences may result in a maladaptive schema such as abandonment, punitive standards, and emotional deprivation (Young et al.,

2003). Segal et al. (1988) proposed that there is a need to reorganise this type of maladaptive schema in therapy; otherwise, the person will be at risk from reactivation when stressed and relapsing into chronic depression is likely to occur.

Schema therapy begins with a series of assessments to educate the client and help them recognise their schemas and their thinking and feelings laid down in childhood causing acute distress in adulthood (The Schema Therapy Institute, www.schemainstitute.co.uk/understanding-schema-therapy/ Retrieved: 22 May 2021). Schema therapy treatment is long-term and incorporates a variety of strategies to facilitate change.

Delivering schema therapy involves techniques based on cognitive, experiential, and behavioural aspects, in addition to a warm and empathic therapeutic relationship (Young et al., 2003). Regarding the cognitive aspect, these strategies are rooted in behaviour therapy and include exploring the pros and cons of a schema, challenging the validity of a schema and facilitating "dialogue between the schema side and the healthy side" (Young et al., 2003, p. 91). Other techniques draw on gestalt psychodrama and experiential imagery techniques (Young et al., 2003). In addition, the client uses flashcards with significant messages established in a therapy session to support them between sessions (Young et al., 2003). For example, an old schema of "I am a failure" might have been reframed to be "I am good enough" and written on the flashcard.

The concept of maladaptive schemas can be incorporated into pluralistic sand-tray therapy. The symbolic process activated by the objects placed in the sand often facilitates the client to explore their experience as a child, linked to their distress as an adult. The client can stay with their distress as they take one step out of their pain due to them taking the observer-experience position, seeing the representation of their experience in the sand tray. The therapist can then help the client work specifically with that schema by suggesting they create a sand display of that dysfunctional pattern and the associated feelings and behaviour. This process may take some time, with the display developing over several sessions. Like the flashcards in schema therapy, the client may eventually construct a new sand display with a reframed schema and the less destructive feelings and behaviours. This transformed schema display is photographed, and the client has a physical image to refer to in between sessions and after therapy.

Mindfulness-based cognitive therapy

Segal et al. (2002) described how mindfulness-based cognitive therapy (MBCT) was developed from a manualised group-skills training to address relapse of severe depression. The rationale based on the view that "individuals who previously experienced episodes of major depression differ from those who have not in the patterns of negative thinking that become activated in mildly depressed moods" (Mark et al., 2008, p. 524).

MBCT psychotherapeutic approach uses CBT methods in collaboration with mindfulness meditative practices and similar psychological strategies (Seligman & Reichenberg, 2014). The aim is to interrupt automatic processes and teach clients to avoid focusing and reacting to these incoming stimuli; to accept and observe these thoughts and feelings without judgment (Felder et al., 2012).

Hofmann et al. (2010) described the process of "decentering" in MBCT, helping clients focus on incoming thoughts and feelings, aiming to accept them without reacting or attaching to them (Hofmann et al., 2010). This method facilitates the client to refrain from self-criticism, rumination, and distress arising from negative thinking. Segal et al. (2002) also note how self-compassion is significant in this process, and Feldman & Kuyken (2011) described how responding to distressing thoughts and feelings with kindness, patience, and empathy is crucial to the process of change.

Kuyken et al. (2010) discussed how some MBCT strategies are used early on in therapy, including mindfulness of the breath, the body scan, and mindful movement. The goal is for the client to step away from habitual negative patterns of thinking, fuelling their depression (Feldman & Kuyken, 2011).

Pluralistic sand-tray therapy can draw upon some of the ideas and methods of MBCT to help meet the client goals. For example, an anxious client might need a strategy to help manage their anxiety outside of therapy. In that case, a mindfulness meditation offered to the client, involving them accepting and observing their anxious thoughts and feelings, can help them avoid self-criticism, rumination, and easing their distress.

This strategy agreed upon with the client and facilitated at the end of a session helps them practice it between sessions when they sense their anxiety beginning to build.

Psychodynamic/Jungian sandplay therapy

Sandplay therapy can be described as a psychodynamic method that is rooted in Jungian theory. As stated earlier, the term "sandplay" was adopted by Jungian scholars to distinguish their approach to that of Lowenfeld's (1979) The world technique. The psychodynamic stance is "primarily concerned with unconscious processes" (Freud, 1963; Howard, 2006, p. 8). The various psychodynamic approaches, including Jungian therapy, "trace their lineage back to Freud and psychoanalysis" (Howard, 2006, p. 8) but have developed their underpinning theoretical stance in different ways. For example, Jungian therapy incorporates the collective unconscious and archetypal universal symbols (Jung, 1969; Kalff, 1980; Kalff, 2003). As Hall and Nordby (1999) described, Jungian theory views the psyche as comprised of consciousness, the personal unconscious and the collective unconscious. Jung (1980) believed that the personal unconscious was the area where memories had been repressed or discarded due to them being either traumatic or insignificant.

The notion of people having "an inner world that has a powerful influence on how we think, feel and behave" (Howard, 2006, p. 9) is also relevant to pluralistic sand-tray therapy. An individual's inner world comprises feelings, memories, and beliefs; partly conscious and partly unconscious is the foundation for the concept of the dynamic phenomenological field (Fleet, 2019) in pluralistic sand-tray therapy. The two sand-tray specific mechanisms of phenomenological anchor and phenomenological hook (Fleet, 2019) were identified as facilitating edge of awareness and unconscious processing that can bring a phenomenological shift as the client engages in the sand-tray process.

Howard (2006) described how the unconscious could be worked with by "the stories we tell, the dreams we relate...slips of the tongue and the use of metaphor and symbolism" (p. 10). In pluralistic sand-tray therapy, it is the use of metaphor and symbolism that is particularly relevant regarding the exploration of the symbolic objects placed in the sand.

Narrative therapy

Narrative therapy became established from family therapy and community work, viewing the person as always "existing within a cultural and historical context" (Sundet & McLeod, 2016, p. 147). Sundet and McLeod (2016) described how narrative therapy understands the person by "careful attention to the use of language, storytelling and dialogue" (p. 155). Madigan (2013) stated, "it is the stories that people tell and hold onto about their lives that shape and determine the meaning they give and how they express their lives" (p. 456).

In narrative therapy, narrative questions are asked to contradict the dominance of the problematic stories in an individual's life (Madigan, 2013). However, narrative questions are never neutral but "state a particular political ideology and location" (p. 456). For example, a female client experiencing anorexia might be asked a question that explores society's expectation for a type of body image regularly communicated by the media and whether the client has ever been able to rebel against such expectations (Madigan, 2013). The aim is to identify the client's strengths and replace the destructive story with an alternative one.

The concept of identity is significant, with social influence being key, as the individual is not viewed as a fixed entity; their identity is thought to be created by the stories they and others tell about who they are (Sundet & McLeod, 2016). Problems occur when the stories conflict with that individual's potential, do not match their day-to-day experience or create disturbance in establishing authentic relationships with others (Sundet & McLeod, 2016).

Brown and Augusta-Scott (2007) discussed the concept of "re-authoring identity" helping a person identify and develop a new story about their identity replacing the destructive dominant narrative with more favourable ones, matching their strengths and resources. In addition, changes to social arrangements and structures in the client's life conducive to the new narrative are encouraged to reside in more supportive and caring environments (Sundet & McLeod, 2016).

In pluralistic sand-tray therapy, the notion of stories can be drawn upon; the client guided to present their stories, using the symbolic objects placed in the sand. The destructive stories related to the client's psychological and emotional distress are explored and replaced with alternative ones. The client can then symbolise the alternative story by creating a new sand display, and their adapted thoughts and feelings explored.

There are similarities between narrative therapy and the pluralistic approach as open dialogue is a crucial feature in both, regarding the client as the expert of their own experience and who can contribute significantly to the therapeutic process (Sundet & McLeod, 2016). However, there are differences between the two approaches. In narrative therapy, the aim is for a "de-centered" relationship. Unlike the pluralistic approach, an authentic relationship between client and therapist is not viewed as significant; instead, the client's connection to other people in their life is a central feature (Sundet & McLeod, 2016).

Practical techniques are used in narrative therapy that can reinforce the adapted stories of a client's life. For example, Ncube and Denborough used creative drawing techniques such as the "tree of life" (Denborough, 2014; Ncube & Denborough, 2007; Ncube, 2006). Working with the metaphor of a tree to symbolise different aspects of the person's life, the different elements of the tree represent different experience. The root represents the person's history, culture, and background; the trunk represents their abilities and the leaves symbolising significant people in their lives, all written down on the tree drawing. Other aspects such as branches represent a person's hopes and dreams, and fruit refers to what they have received and given to others. The aim is for the person to share their stories with the listener asking questions to help establish alternative stories that incorporate their strengths, skills, and hopes.

The "tree of life" exercise can be incorporated into a structured pluralistic sand-tray therapy session if the client is happy to work that way. Often it can help a client connect with the process if they can touch and work with the sand by using their fingers. In this exercise, the client might outline a tree in the sand and select objects to represent their experience. The exercise is only a starting point to help the client begin exploring their phenomenological experience, and the process of touch can bring profound connection, often facilitating edge of awareness and unconscious processing, leading to phenomenological shift as they recreate their story.

References

Baker, N. (2012). Experiential Person-Centred Therapy. In Pete Sanders (Ed.). *The Tribes of the Person-Centred Nation: An Introduction to She Schools of Therapy Related to the Person-Centred Approach.* Chapter 4, pp. 67–94. Monmouth: PCCS Books.

Beck, A. T. (1964). Thinking and depression: II. Theory and therapy: *Archives of General Psychiatry*. 10, 561–571.

Beck, A. T., Rush, A. J., Shaw, B. F., & Emery, G. (1979). *Cognitive Therapy for Depression*. New York: The Guildford Press.

Berg, I. K. (1994). *Family-Based Services: A Solution-Focused Approach*, New York: W.W. Norton and Company, Inc.

Berg, I. K., & de Shazer, S. (1993). Making Numbers Talk. In Friedman, S. *The New Language of Change: Constructive Collaboration in Psychotherapy*. New York: Guildford Press.

Boucher, T. (2016). Cognitive Behavioural Approaches and Pluralism. In Mick Cooper and Windy Dryden (Eds.). *The Handbook of Pluralistic Counselling and Psychotherapy*. Chapter 9, pp. 108–121. London: Sage.

Boyes, C. (2008). *Need to Know? Cognitive Behavioural Therapy. Think Better. Be Happier*. London: HarperCollins Publishers.

Brown, C., & Augusta-Scott, T. (eds). (2007). *Narrative Therapy: Making Meaning, Making Lives*. Thousand Oaks, CA: Sage. ISBN 978-1412909877

Bugental, J. F. T. (1964). The third force in psychology. *The Journal of Humanistic Psychology*. 4(1), 19–26.

Carter, J. D., McIntosh, V. V., Jordan, J., Porter, R. J., Frampton, C. M., & Joyce. P. R. (2013). Psychotherapy for depression: A randomized clinical trial comparing schema therapy and cognitive behavior therapy. *Journal of Affective Disorders*. 151, 500–505.

Cooper, M. (2012). Existentially Informed Person-Centred Therapy. In Pete Sanders (Ed.). *The Tribes of the Person-Centred Nation: An Introduction to She Schools of Therapy Related to the Person-Centred Approach*. Chapter 6, pp. 131–160. Monmouth: PCCS Books.

Corcoran, J. & Pillai, V. (2007). A review of the research on solution focused therapy. *British Journal of Social Work*. 39(2), 234–242.

Denborough, D. (2014). *Retelling the stories of our lives. Everyday narrative Therapy to Draw Inspiration and Transform Experience*. New York: W.W. Norton.

de Shazer, S. (1985). *Keys to Solution in Brief Therapy*. New York: W.W. Norton & Company.

de Shazer, S. (1988). *Clues: Investigating Solutions in Brief Therapy*. New York: W.W. Norton & Company.

de Shazer, S. (1994). *Words Were Originally Magic*. New York: Norton.

de Shazer, S., Berg, I. K., Lipchik, E., Nunnally, E., Molnar, A., Gingerich, W., & Weiner-Davis, M. (1986). Brief therapy: focused solution development. *Family Process*. 25(2), 207–221.

Elliott, R., Watson, R, C., Goldman, R. N., & Greenberg, L. S. (2004). *Learning Emotion-Focused Therapy: The Process-Experiential Approach to Change*. Washington, DC: American Psychological Association.

Ellis, A. (1962). *Reason and Emotion in Psychotherapy*. New York: Lyle Stuart.

Elliott, R. (2012). Emotion-focuses therapy. In P. Sanders (Ed.). *The tribes of the person-centred nation*. (2nd ed.) (pp. 103–130). Ross-on-Wye: PCCS Books.

Farrell, J. M., Reiss, N., & Shaw, I. A. (2014). *The Schema Therapy Clinician's Guide A Complete Resource for Building and Delivering Individual, Group and Integrated Schema Mode Treatment Programs*. Chichester, West Sussex: John Wiley & Sons, Ltd.

Felder, J. N., Dimidjian, S., & Segal, Z. (2012). Collaboration in mindfulness-based cognitive therapy. *Journal of Clinical Psychology.* 68(2), 179–186. doi:10.1002/jclp.21832. PMID 23616298.

Feldman. C., & Kuyken, W. (2011) Compassion in the landscape of suffering, *Contemporary Buddhism*, 12(1), 143–155. DOI: 10.1080/14639947.2011.564831

Fleet, D. (2019). *Transformation hidden in the sand: developing a theoretical framework using a sand-tray intervention with adult clients.* Doctoral thesis. Staffordshire University. Stoke-on-Trent. Available from Ethos STORE – Staffordshire Online Repository. https://eprints.staffs.ac.uk/id/eprint/5763

Freeth, R. (2007). *Humanising Psychiatry and Mental Health Care: The Challenge of the Person-centred Approach.* Oxford: Radcliffe Publishing.

Freud, S. (1963). *General Psychological Theory. Papers on Metapsychology.* New York: Collier Books-Macmillan Publishing Company.

Fuller, M. (1810–1850). US Transcendentalist author & editor. https://in.pinterest.com Retrieved 27 April 2021.

Gendlin, E. T. (1969). *Focusing-Orientated Psychotherapy.* New York: Guilford Press.

Gendlin, E. T. (1981). *Focusing.* (2nd edition). New York: Bantam Books.

Gendlin, E. T. (1984). The Clients' Client: The Edge of Awareness. In R. F. Levant & J. M. Shlien (eds.). *Client-Centered Therapy and the Person-Centered Approach: New Directions in Theory, Research, and Practice.* (pp. 76–107). New York: Praeger.

Gendlin, E. T. (1996). Focusing Orientated Psychotherapy: A manual of the experiential method. New York, NY10012: The Guildford Press.

Gilbert, P., & Irons, C. (2005). Focused Therapies and Compassionate Mind Training for Shame and Self-attacking. In P. Gilbert (Ed.). *Compassion: Conceptualisations, research and use in psychotherapy.* (pp. 263–325). London: Routledge.

Gilbert, P. (2007). The Evolution of Shame as a Marker for Relationship Security. In J. L. Tracy, R. W. Robins & J. P. Tangney (Eds.). The self-conscious emotions: Theory and research. (pp. 283–309). New York: Guildford Press.

Gilbert, P. (2009a). *The Compassionate Mind: A New Approach to the Challenges of Life.* London, UK: Constable & Robinson.

Gilbert, P. (2009b). Introducing compassion-focused therapy. *Advances in Psychiatric Treatment.* 15 (3): 199–208. doi:10.1192/apt.bp.107.005264.

Gilbert, P. (2010). *Compassion Focused Therapy: The DBT Distinctive Features Series.* London, UK: Routledge.

Greenberg, L. S. (1979). Resolving splits: Use of the two-chair technique. *Psychotherapy: Theory, Research & Practice.* 16(3), 316–324. doi.org/10.1037/h0085895

Greenberg, L. S., Rice, L. N., & Elliott, R. (1993). *Facilitating Emotional Change: The Moment-by-moment Process.* New York: Guildford Press.

Greenberg, L. S. (2004). Emotion-focused therapy. *Clinical Psychology & Psychotherapy, 11,* 3–16.

Hall, C. & Nordby, V. (1999). *The Primer of Jungian Psychology.* New York: Meridian

Hanley, T., Scott, A., & Winter, L. A. (2016). Humanistic Approaches and Pluralism. In Mick Cooper and Windy Dryden (Eds.). *The Handbook of Pluralistic Counselling and Psychotherapy.* Chapter 8, pp. 95–107. London: Sage.

Hofmann, S. G., Sawyer, A. T., & Fang, A. (2010). The Empirical Status of the "New Wave" of Cognitive Behavioral Therapy. *Psychiatric Clinics of North America.* 33(3), 701–710. doi:10.1016/j.psc.2010.04.006. PMC 2898899. PMID 20599141.

Homeyer, L. E., & Sweeney, D. S. (2011). *Sandtray Therapy: A Practical Manual.* 2nd ed. London: Routledge.

Howard, S. (2006). *Psychodynamic Counselling in a Nutshell.* London: Sage.

Jung. C. G. (1969). *Archetypes and the Collective Unconscious. Collected Works of C. C. Jung.* Volume 9 (Part 1). Princeton, NJ: Princeton University Press.

Jung, C. G. (1980). *The Archetypes and the Collective Unconscious.* Princeton, NJ: Princeton University Press. (Original work published 1959.)

Kalff, D. M. (1980). *Sandplay.* Boston: Sigo Press.

Kalff, D. (2003). *Sandplay: A Psychotherapeutic Approach to the Psyche.* Cloverdale, CA: Temenos PR.

Kim, J. S. (2008). Examining the effectiveness of solution focused brief therapy: A metaanalysis. *Research on Social Work Practice.* 18(2), 107–116.

Kolts, R. (2016). *CFT Made Simple: A Clinician's Guide to Practicing Compassion-Focused Therapy.* Oakland, CA: New Harbinger Publications. ISBN 9781626253094. OCLC 914290386.

Kuyken, W., Watkins, E., Holden, E., White, K., Taylor, R. S., Byford, S., Evans, A., Radford, S., Teasdale, J. D., & Dalgleish, T. (2010). *Behaviour Research and Therapy.* 48, 1105–1112.

Lowenfeld, M. (1979). *The World Technique.* London: Allen & Unwin.

Madigan, S. (2013). Narrative Therapy. In Davies, M. (Ed.). *The Blackwell Companion to Social Work.* (pp. 455–457). United Kingdom: John Wiley & Sons.

Mark, J., Williams, G., Russell, I., & Russell, D. (2008). Mindfulness-based cognitive therapy: Further issues in current evidence and future research. *Journal of Consulting and Clinical Psychology.* 76(3), 524–529.

McMillan, M. (2004). *The Person-Centred Approach to Therapeutic Change.* London: Sage.

Mearns, D., & Thorne, B. (1999). *Person-Centred Counselling in Action.* (2nd ed.). London: Sage.

Merry, T. (2004). Classical client-centred therapy. In P. Sanders, (Ed.). *The Tribes of the Person-Centred Nation: An Introduction to the Schools of Therapy Related to the Person-Centred Approach*, (2012, pp. 21–44). Ross-on-Wye: PCCS Books.

Ncube, N. (2006). The tree of life project. Using narrative ideas in work with vulnerable children in southern Africa. *International Journal of Narrative Therapy & Community Work.* (1), 3–16.

Ncube, N. (2017). *Tree of life. Practitioners Guide.* Johannesburg: Phola.

Ncube – Milo, N., & Denborough D. (2007). *Tree of Life. The Mainstreaming Psycho Social Care and Support: A Manual for Facilitators.* Johannesburg: Regional Psychosocial Support Initiative REPSSI.

Piaget, J. (1952). *The Origins of Intelligence in Children.* (M. Cook, Trans.). New York, NY: W. W. Norton & Co. https://doi.org/10.1037/11494-000

Perls, F. S. (1969). *Gestalt Therapy Verbatim.* Moab, UT: Real People Press.

Perls, F. S. (1973). *The Gestalt Approach and Eye Witness to Therapy* (1973). Ben Lomond: California. Science & Behavior Books. ISBN 0-8314-0034-X

Perls, F., Hefferline, R., & Goodman, P. (1994). *Gestalt Therapy/Excitement and Growth in the Human Personality.* London: Souvenir Press.

Purton, C. (2012). Focusing-Orientated Therapy. In Pete Sanders (Ed.). *The Tribes of the Person-Centred Nation: An Introduction to She Schools of Therapy Related to the Person-Centred Approach.* Chapter 3, pp. 47–69. Monmouth: PCCS Books.

Rogers, C. R. (1951). *Client-Centered Therapy: Its Current Practice, Implications and Theory.* London: Constable.

Rogers, C. R. (1957). The necessary and sufficient conditions of therapeutic personality change. *Journal of Consulting Psychology, 21*, 95–103.

Rogers, C. R. (1961). *On Becoming a Person: A Therapist's View of Psychotherapy.* London: Constable.

Rogers, C. R. (1980). *A Way of Being.* Boston, New York: Houghton Mifflin Company.

Sanders, P. (2004; 2012). *The Tribes of the Person-Centred Nation: An Introduction to She Schools of Therapy Related to the Person-Centred Approach.* Monmouth: PCCS Books.

Segal, Z. V., Hood, J. E., Shaw, B. F., & Higgins, E. T. (1988). A structural analysis of the self-schema construct in major depression. *Cognitive Therapy and Research.* 12 (5), 471–485.

Segal, Z. V., & Williams, J. M. G., & Teasdale, J. D. (2002). *Mindfulness-Based Cognitive Therapy for Depression: A New Approach to Preventing Relapse.* New York: The Guildford Press.

Seligman, L. W., & Reichenberg, L. W. (2014). *Theories of Counseling and Psychotherapy.* 4th Edition. London, UK: Prentice Hall.

Stalker, C.A., Levene, J., & Coady, N.F. (1999). Solution focused brief therapy – one model fits all? Families in Society: *Journal of Contemporary Human Services.* 80(5), 468–483.

Stevens, C. (2004). Playing in the sand. *The British Gestalt Journal*, 13(1), 18–23. Retrieved from www.psychotherapynottingham.com/Pages/Playing_in_th_Sand. html

Sundet, R., & McLeod, J. (2016). Narrative approaches and pluralism. In M. Cooper & W. Dryden (Eds.). *Handbook of Pluralistic Counselling and Psychotherapy.* (pp. 158–170). London: Sage.

Taylor, E. R. (2009). Sandtray and solution-focused therapy. *International Journal of Play Therapy, 18*(1), 56–68.

Whelton, W. J., & Greenberg, L. (2005). Emotion in Self-criticism. Personality and Individual Differences, 38(7), 1538–1595.

Young, J. (1990). *Cognitive Therapy for Personality Disorders: A Schema-Focused Approach.* Professional Resource Press, Florida.

Young, J. E., Klosoko, J. S., & Weisharr, M. E. (2003). *Schema Therapy: A Practitioner's Guide.* New York: The Guildford Press.

Index

For Product Safety Concerns and Information please contact our EU
representative GPSR@taylorandfrancis.com
Taylor & Francis Verlag GmbH, Kaufingerstraße 24, 80331 München, Germany